'This practical follow-up to the authors' earlier work on finding meaning in dementia through spiritual reminiscence is most welcome. It encourages small group leaders to develop and employ the requisite empathetic and communication skills, and offers a course based on six topics that have proved fruitful in helping those attending to feel that they have really been listened to.'

– Revd Dr Albert Jewell, editor of Spirituality and Personhood in Dementia *and of the Christian Council on Ageing's Dementia Newsletter, Visiting Research Fellow at Glyndwyr University*

'This helpful handbook shows that spirituality is not the province of experts. Carers can ask: "who is this person?" Step by step strategies prompt discussion of grief, guilt, fears, regrets, joys; also uncovering the dreaded issues of death and dying. The authors' central message is that symbols may be more important than words and engaging with life's meaning better than medication.'

– Rosalie Hudson, Associate Professor (honorary), School of Nursing, University of Melbourne and Adjunct Associate Professor, Charles Sturt University

'An outstanding book that demonstrates spiritual reminiscence can be highly successful in giving meaning, hope and perspective to people living with dementia in ways not traditionally thought possible. This is an invaluable resource for facilitators, providing guidance for each session. It challenges the facilitator to explore their own spirituality to ensure they are able to journey with others.'

– Elizabeth Pringle, former General Manager Operations Australian Aged Care Quality Agency (AACQA) and consultant, Improvement Matters

Facilitating Spiritual Reminiscence for Older People with Dementia

A Learning Guide

Elizabeth MacKinlay
and Corinne Trevitt

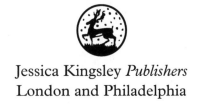

Jessica Kingsley *Publishers*
London and Philadelphia

First published in 2015
by Jessica Kingsley Publishers
73 Collier Street
London N1 9BE, UK
and
400 Market Street, Suite 400
Philadelphia, PA 19106, USA

www.jkp.com

Library of Congress Cataloging in Publication Data
MacKinlay, Elizabeth, 1940-
  Facilitating spiritual reminiscence for older people with dementia : a learning guide / Elizabeth MacKinlay and Corinne Trevitt.
    pages cm
  Includes bibliographical references.
  ISBN 978-1-84905-573-4 (alk. paper)
  1. Senile dementia--Patients--Care. 2. Senile dementia--Patients--Religious life. 3. Senile dementia--Patients--Pastoral counseling of. 4. Reminiscing in old age--Therapeutic use. 5. Spirituality. I. Trevitt, Corinne. II. Title.
  RC524.M27 2015
  616.8'3--dc23
                            2014047205

British Library Cataloguing in Publication Data
A CIP catalogue record for this book is available from the British Library

ISBN 978 1 84905 573 4
eISBN 978 1 78450 018 4

Printed and bound in the United States

Contents

Acknowledgements

The learning guide could not have been completed without the support of the following funding groups:

- research pilot: University of Canberra Collaborative Grant

- research project: Australian Research Council (ARC) Linkage Grant

- trial of the learning guide: J.O. and J.R. Wicking Trust.

The authors would like to extend their thanks to all the older people with dementia who have shared their lives with us. It has been a privilege and joy to hear their stories.

We would also like to thank the aged care facilities that supported and contributed to these grants and participated in the Spiritual Reminiscence Project from 2003–2005:

- Anglican Retirement Community Services Canberra and Merimbula

- Wesley Gardens Uniting Care Ageing, Sydney

- Mirinjani Village, Uniting Care Ageing, Canberra.

Preface

Over more than a decade we have spent many hours listening and speaking to older people who have dementia. They have shared about their lives, where they find meaning; and about their hopes, fears and regrets. This has come about primarily through a project titled 'Finding meaning in the experience of dementia: The place of spiritual reminiscence work'. It has been both a privilege and a revelation to listen to the stories and to help these people explore emotional and spiritual issues through spiritual reminiscence.

What is spiritual reminiscence?

Spiritual reminiscence is a particular way of communication that acknowledges the person as a spiritual being and seeks to engage the person in a more meaningful and personal way. It focuses on the person and their emotional and spiritual being rather than on cognitive losses. Research has demonstrated that interactions among those with dementia are increased following group work in spiritual reminiscence for a period of up to six months (MacKinlay and Trevitt, 2005, 2012). Spiritual reminiscence in small groups also helps older people with dementia bond and develop friendships in a way that is often otherwise difficult to nurture in aged care facilities. These people have often lost most of the important relationships of their lives, and their communication difficulties make it harder for them to meet and get to know others in the new environment of residential aged care.

While analyzing the data for this project we noticed that some facilitators of spiritual reminiscence were more skilled at assisting people with dementia to communicate within a small group than others. So we carefully considered what factors were important in facilitating, or inhibiting the group process. The result was the development of this learning guide to assist facilitators who work with small groups of people who have dementia. This guide ensures that everyone wanting to use spiritual reminiscence as a way to communicate with those with or without dementia can develop appropriate skills.

This guide may be used with the book: *Finding Meaning in the Experience of Dementia: The Place of Spiritual Reminiscence Work* (MacKinlay and Trevitt, 2012) which provides the theory and background involved with the research of this project, also published by Jessica Kingsley Publishers. We hope that you enjoy working through this learning guide. The information you gain and the skills you develop help you to communicate in a meaningful way with all older people.

Throughout this guide there are 'Important Point' and 'Think About' boxes. These highlight important parts of the narrative and guide you to consider more deeply some of the issues discussed. You may wish to compile a journal of your reflections about using the guide based on the 'Think About' points. A reflective journal will also help you to gather you thoughts and reflect on facilitating a spiritual reminiscence group.

The impact of spiritual reminiscence groups

The following summary of the major outcomes of the original project is from the perspective of the pastoral carers on behalf of the residents involved in the ARC Linkage research project:

- The residents benefited from meeting together as a group – especially the six month group as opposed to the six week one. They eventually knew each other well and formed friendships, some of which have lasted since 2003 and must have made a difference to the quality of their lives.

- They eagerly came to the group each week, greeting each other cheerfully and chatting together before the formal questions began. This was not the norm for many activities with these residents, as they are often not sure what is going on.

- They had others to talk to in the rather large number of people who assembled for meals or other activities in the lounge/dining room, and I noticed that the members of the group were more likely to chat to new residents.

- On two occasions a hurt from many years ago was raised and I was able to talk privately with that person later.

- The residents from the group developed greater confidence than before and seemed better able to cope with their daily activities.

- Without exception their relatives or guardians were enthusiastic about their taking part in the study, saw it as beneficial to them and were happy to think the results would help others.

(MacKinlay and Trevitt, 2005)

Comments at the completion of the weekly groups

The following are some comments made by group members at the completion of the spiritual reminiscence groups.

Amy: Does you good to remember too – things that we've talked about – now we've talked them over – they come back more easily – and you can visualise them again.

Amy: Perhaps I can't put my – perhaps what I like to say – but it has been a wonderful help and company and I'm certainly am going to miss it on a Friday afternoon.

Facilitator: Why do you like coming?

Peter: Well I like the interchange of talk and getting to know more people.

Facilitator:	Do you like discussing things?
Peter:	Yes I do. Not that I am very good at it, but I just like listening to people. People's ideas on certain subjects.

Frequently, participants in the groups said that the process of spiritual reminiscence allowed them to talk about issues that were important to them in a more meaningful way that was not generally on offer in an aged care facility.

The majority of participants in the groups had at least moderate levels of dementia, and sufficient cognitive decline to need residential care (for more details of the participants see MacKinlay and Trevitt, 2012). The exchanges among participants demonstrated that these older people with dementia had not lost their sense of humour and many of the exchanges had a background of laughter. Sometimes humour arose as group members discussed issues around memory loss and dying, and this was probably a means of lightening or diffusing the topic. Death is yet another topic that facilitators need to feel comfortable with speaking of in the groups.

Participants spoke to each other and developed friendships within the facility as a result of the interactions during the spiritual reminiscence group. Often when topics were raised there was a lot of discussion among the participants about the issue. This sometimes depended on the length of time the group had been established – and it was certainly evident in the 24 week groups that the level of trust that developed allowed frequent verbal interchanges.

Learning outcomes for the spiritual reminiscence program

On completion of the learning guide you will be able to:

- differentiate between reminiscence and spiritual reminiscence

- explain the role of spiritual reminiscence as an aspect of spiritual care in the holistic care of older people who have dementia

- demonstrate the specific communication skills required when interacting with a person with dementia

- facilitate spiritual reminiscence groups for older people with and without dementia.

This learning guide is designed to assist you to develop skills to undertake spiritual reminiscence with older people who have dementia. Although this learning guide is designed specifically for interactions with older adults with dementia, these skills are transferable and can be used with any group of older adults.

The guide is divided into two parts. Part 1, is entitled 'Learning about working with people who have dementia: Story, spirituality and spiritual reminiscence'. It contains necessary background to working effectively with people who have dementia and especially, the process of reminiscence and spiritual reminiscence. Part 2, containing the weekly sessions of spiritual reminiscence, provides the 'how to' guide for facilitating spiritual reminiscence. Elizabeth and Corinne provide this guide to meet your needs for learning more about spiritual reminiscence and to give you the skills and confidence to facilitate a group.

Part 1

Learning about working with people who have dementia: Story, spirituality and spiritual reminiscence

Chapter 1

Spiritual care

In the day-to-day care of older people with dementia it is often easy to slip into the process of physical care at the expense of psychosocial, emotional and spiritual care. Indeed, in the midst of a busy day when there are staff shortages and older people with high level care needs, it is often the physical needs that receive priority and are taken care of first – any time left over can perhaps be devoted to other aspects of care. However, if we believe that each person deserves to be treated with dignity and care, then we need to provide holistic care. Holistic care means recognizing and addressing physical, social, psychological, emotional and spiritual needs of older people.

Spiritual needs are just as important as other needs, in fact one manager in aged care has said that about three quarters of her work involved matters of grief, guilt and fear. These are certainly issues of the spiritual dimension.

Spiritual needs are just as important as other needs.

Good person-centred care takes into account the spiritual as well as the emotional, psychosocial and physical needs of people. However, we have found in recent work with activities in residential aged care (Byrne and MacKinlay, 2012), that often, the basic practice of person-centred care, that we thought was well established, did not happen, especially when staff were adding new skills to their already established skills. Further, we have found that some staff still work from the premise that when a person's cognitive status declines, communication should be restricted to factual and concrete examples, which is far from true. People with little cognitive function can and do respond positively to emotional and spiritual input. In fact they may respond to the spiritual and emotional when they are no longer able to respond cognitively. Our attitudes to people with failing cognitive abilities can have a real impact on either supporting or limiting interaction with people who have dementia. Spiritual and emotional care are closely associated with effective person-centred care. But, having said that, we need to look at what spirituality really is.

What is spirituality? Is it different from religion?

Describing the spiritual domain has always been difficult. Even now, when there seems to be a rising awareness of the spiritual in society there has been little agreement on what is the spiritual domain; if everyone has it, if it ought to be addressed, and if so by whom, and how.

However, it would be fair to say that spirituality is about meaning in life and relationship, and as such it is a critical part of what it is to be human (MacKinlay, 2012). Some people see religion and spirituality as being the same. Others say that there is no relationship between religion and spirituality. In this learning guide, it is maintained that religion and spirituality are connected, but that while some people do not practise a religion, all do have a spiritual dimension.

Spirituality is about meaning in life and is mediated through:
- *relationship (with God and/or others)*
- *the arts*
- *the environment or creation and involves human creativity and imagination*
- *religion (religion takes in all aspects of spirituality).*

(MacKinlay, 2012, p.16)

When we talk about spirituality we are not referring to religiousness although of course, religion is part of spirituality for those who have a religious faith. Often spiritual care is not seen as a priority because the older person does not declare a religion or go to church. A better way to think about spirituality is to imagine that spirituality is an umbrella. Religion comes in under this umbrella and is one way to express this spirituality. Figure 1.1, based on MacKinlay 2006 (modified), helps to illustrate this concept.

There has recently been an increasing interest in studying the spiritual dimension. It is suggested (MacKinlay, 2001, 2006) that issues of a spiritual nature become more important as people age. Findings from a recent study of baby-boomer ageing show the importance of spirituality in later life (MacKinlay and Burns, unpublished study 2013), with spirituality associated with promoting mental and physical health and lower anxiety about ageing. It also found that baby boomers were not necessarily affiliated with religious organizations but had higher levels of spirituality.

There are many definitions of spirituality. The following definition arises from work undertaken by Elizabeth MacKinlay. She defines spirituality as:

That which lies at the core of each person's being, an essential dimension which brings meaning to life. Constituted not only by religious practices, but understood more broadly, as relationship with God, however God or ultimate meaning is perceived by the person, and in relationship with other people. (MacKinlay, 2001, p.52)

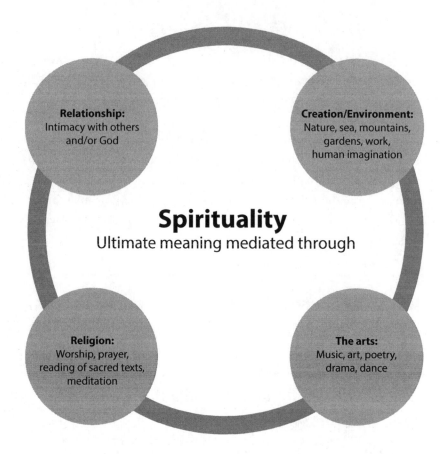

Figure 1.1: Spirituality and religion (adapted from MacKinlay, 2006)

What is spiritual care?

Providing spiritual care is about tapping into the concept of spirituality – core meaning, deepest life-meaning and relationship. For some older people it may be expressed in a relationship with God or higher being, for others it could be expressed through nature, the environment and/or family and friends. It is what lies at the centre, the heart of our being and is from where we respond to all of life. Anger, hate, love, forgiveness and hope come from the heart.

Spiritual care in multi-cultural and multi-faith communities

Increasingly in western countries, care is being provided within a multi-cultural and multi-faith environment. Everyone associated with aged care needs first to be aware of their own spirituality and faith perspective, before they are able to meet the needs of others who may come from a different faith background. This 'self-knowing' is an important part of providing spiritual care.

If we recognize the spiritual dimension in ageing and want to really make a difference for older persons in need of care, the spiritual dimension must be recognized as a real dimension of holistic care.

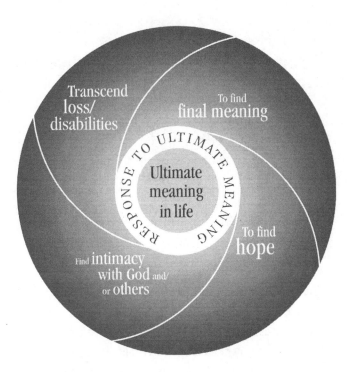

Figure 1.2: A Model of Spiritual Tasks and Process of Ageing (MacKinlay, 2006, p.23)

This model (Figure 1.2) provides a framework for understanding spiritual processes in ageing. The model in this learning guide is a generic model based on people with and without a religious faith perspective. For a model of spiritual tasks and process of ageing for Christians, see MacKinlay, 2006; other models for major faith groups are being developed. The model used in this learning guide centres on the human search for meaning, and the associated responses to perceived meaning; the other tasks involve the development of transcendence (the ability to triumph over the psychosocial, physical and spiritual challenges of ageing) moving from provisional to final life-meanings, finding intimacy and finding hope. In the context of spiritual reminiscence it has a focus on story and finding meaning through the story. This model allows for continued spiritual growth and development until the end of life. It also suggests opportunities for spiritual assessment and intervention (a spiritual assessment form can be found in MacKinlay, 2006, pp.246–252).

The Model of Spiritual Tasks and Process of Ageing

First, a word of explanation about the model. A model can be helpful in understanding what is happening in a situation. It can enhance our ability to see patterns and identify opportunities for change and interventions where these are needed.

The word 'task' is used in this context to explain the potential spiritual changes that can take place, most often in the later years of life. We have added the term 'process' to the model, as when Elizabeth first developed the model of spiritual tasks (MacKinlay, 2001), some thought that it was simply tasks to be done, ticked off, and completed. However, the model is not only about individual and isolated tasks, but a process that can potentially last until the end of life, with spiritual growth and development continuing unless blocked in some way.

At least some of the spiritual tasks and processes of ageing are related to physical and mental changes that occur in later life. These changes involve losses frequently encountered in ageing such as, loss of relationships, place of dwelling and/or health. In particular, bodily changes, living with chronic diseases and energy loss are more likely to stimulate thoughts of mortality and stimulate transcendence. The Model of Spiritual Tasks and Process of Ageing is described below.

The first two spiritual tasks of ageing are to find ultimate meaning in life, while the second is to respond to that ultimate meaning. These lie at the heart of what it is to be human.

Ultimate meaning

What brings greatest meaning and purpose to each individual is the starting point for that person. For example, if core or deepest meaning comes through relationship with loved ones, it is important to know this, especially if there has been a loss of relationship through death. Meaning is at the centre of what it is to be human and loss of meaning can be an important factor in grief and depression. These ideas will be explored more fully as part of the weekly spiritual reminiscence process.

Meaning is at the centre of what it is to be human.

This response is a reaching out from our depth, from our deepest thoughts, beliefs and feelings to otherness and to others. In the studies of spirituality of older people (MacKinlay, 2001, 2006), a range of responses was found. If art, or music, or environment were central sources of meaning, then the person would respond to meaning through this. If God is central in meaning, then worship, prayer, reading of sacred scriptures or meditation are likely to be means of response.

Even in secular societies, the use of symbols and rituals binds people together in finding the meaning of major life events. Finding meaning is crucially important in such events as sudden loss of life, floods, bush fires and other natural disasters. In past centuries, religious bodies were central in helping people find meaning through worship and ritual; now in secular societies, the human need for meaning through ritual and symbol has not diminished.

This need can be addressed by engaging with the spiritual in creative and imaginative ways. Religious services of worship remain important to those who hold a religious faith. Rituals and symbols help people to connect with meaning, to respond appropriately to loss and to begin to grieve, or to forgive or to seek reconciliation.

The use of meaningful symbols and rituals supports hope and healing for those who participate.

The remaining spiritual tasks of ageing are finding relationship and connectedness, which is expressed in Figure 1.2 as finding intimacy with God and/or others (often in the face of loss of important relationships), finding final meaning through story (the focus of spiritual reminiscence), dealing with issues of vulnerability expressed in Figure 1.2 as transcend loss/disability leading to self-transcendence and finally, hope versus fear.

Spiritual care and spiritual reminiscence

Spiritual care is very important to quality of life, health and well-being, particularly in later life. One important way of addressing the spiritual needs of older people is through spiritual reminiscence. Spiritual reminiscence allows people to talk about the things in their lives that have held great meaning for them. It also gives them permission to remember past events over which they may have felt angry, sad or guilty, or even regretted. It can help people to reframe events that occurred in the past and come to new understandings and perhaps a sense of peace.

The first part of enhancing spiritual care is to raise spiritual awareness among those who work with older people, including aged care staff (MacKinlay, 2001). Some people say that issues of spirituality are very private issues and should not be raised. However, we have found that numbers of older people with dementia do want to talk about these issues (MacKinlay, 2001, 2006; MacKinlay and Trevitt, 2012). Some want to review their lives and perhaps wish to share with one or more people how they feel about the kinds of lives they have lived.

Providing spiritual care and self-awareness of staff members

Learning new skills in providing care is valuable, but even more valuable, and a first step to being able to provide high quality spiritual care is spiritual self-awareness of the care provider. As a short guide to raising self-awareness please complete the short exercise in the box on the following page.

> How aware are you of your spirituality?
>
> How comfortable are you speaking to others about spirituality?

It is important that those who work with people who have dementia, especially in providing spiritual care, have examined their own spirituality. This is privileged work, and not an opportunity for proselytizing.

The following exercise is valuable in coming to a greater understanding of your own beliefs and values. It should at least be worked through by each person, before preparing to facilitate spiritual reminiscence. If possible it is valuable to share your understanding of the spiritual dimension with a small group of other people: it might be work colleagues or a workshop, or a faith community.

The following exercise should be done by the individual before sharing with others.

Speaking to others about spirituality

Before we go any further, take time to explore your own spiritual core.

Think about and answer the following:

- What gives you most meaning in your life?
- Looking back over your life so far:
  - » What has made you feel happy or sad?
  - » What has brought you joy?
  - » Do you have any regrets?
  - » Do you have any fears for the future?
- What or who is most important in your life?
- Do you have any religious or spiritual practices that are important to you?

How do you feel about providing spiritual care for people from different cultures and faiths and those who may or may not have a religious faith?

Chapter 2

Dementia

Dementia is a condition feared by many people, no matter what their age. Even diseases such as cancer and disabilities such as stroke or arthritis do not strike the same fears as dementia. In a study of older independent living people, it was identified as a fear by one third of participants (MacKinlay, 2001) with one participant describing that she did not want to be 'off her legs and out of her mind' (p.143). Relatives often describe their loved one as 'having already gone' or that they experience death twice – once as a result of memory loss and then again when the person truly dies. A number of authors support this view that the person is 'gone' (Porter, 2002 and De Baggio, 2003). However, other literature supports the view that the person remains, even if in a different way, (Killick, 2006; Kitwood 1997). An important understanding of this newer view of dementia is from Hughes, Louw and Sabat: 'people with dementia have to be understood in terms of relationships, not because this is all that is left to them, but because this is characteristic of all our lives' (2006, p.35).

Dementia is responsible for progressive cognitive and functional impairment over a period of years, with great cost to individuals, families and the community. As a person ages there is an increasing chance of developing dementia – although dementia is not a normal part of ageing. In Australia 1 in 10 people over 65 has dementia and 3 in 10 of those over 85 years old (Australian Institute of Health and Welfare, 2012). These figures are similar across the world (Ferri *et al*, 2005). In residential aged care facilities more than 50 per cent of residents are identified as having dementia (AIHW, 2012). While there is continuing research into both the causes of dementia and pharmacological cures, the greatest need presently is to find ways to enhance quality of life for those diagnosed with dementia. This means there needs to be an emphasis on understanding the world of the person with dementia and on communication that can tap into the 'inner core of being' of the person with dementia.

In the early stages the person may notice some word finding problems and short-term memory loss but can still use strategies to overcome these losses. Stokes (2010) describes in detail the story of a woman who was just managing to keep her household together by writing lists of everything that she had to do each day. Her family noticed changes in her behaviour but because of her frantic list making were unable to 'catch her out'.

In the mid and later stages of dementia this memory loss becomes more obvious and the person will experience difficulty maintaining tasks of daily living, driving, shopping, managing finances and living independently. In the later stages self-care tasks such as dressing, bathing, eating and drinking become impossible and the person requires full-time care.

We tend to think about those with dementia as being all the same with memory loss being the predominant problem. But each person with dementia experiences the changes brought about by dementia in a different way, thus care always needs to be individualized. We need to meet each person as they are, and acknowledge them as an individual human being, regardless of cognitive abilities. Practices that work for one person may cause agitation and discomfort in another. For this reason, dementia remains one of the most challenging syndromes affecting older people.

When we talk about dementia we often immediately think of Alzheimer's disease but this is just one of about a hundred different conditions that are characterized by loss of cognitive function (AIHW, 2012). These types of dementia are differentiated by their presentation, the person's previous medical history and often by the types of symptoms that are the most prevalent. Alzheimer's disease remains the most common type of dementia accounting for about 50–75 per cent of all dementias (AIHW, 2012). The other most common types of dementia include vascular dementia (20–30%), fronto-temporal dementia (5–10%), and dementia with Lewy bodies (up to 5%) (AIHW, 2012). The number of people worldwide who were estimated to have some type of dementia in 2005 was 24 million people (Ferri *et al.*, 2005). This will continue to increase with the ageing of populations.

Dementia is a leading cause of disability in people aged 65 and over, responsible for one year in every six years of disability burden. It is the third greatest source of health and residential care spending (Access Economics, 2009). A similar picture is seen in the USA with more than five million Americans currently believed to have Alzheimer's disease and expected to rise to 15 million by 2050 (Alzheimer's Disease Research, 2011). In the UK there are currently 750,000 people with dementia, with 16,000 younger people having been diagnosed. Sixty-four per cent of people living in care homes have some form of dementia (Alzheimer's Society, 2011).

Seventy per cent of people over age of eighty-five will not develop dementia. (Consistent with figures from Access Economics, 2009, Australia; Alzheimer's Disease Research, 2011, USA and Alzheimer's Society, 2011, UK.)

It can be helpful for carers though to be aware of some of the differences in the different types. For example, those with Alzheimer's tend to have less depression than those with vascular dementia; fronto-temporal dementia causes more verbal outbursts and inappropriate activities; paranoid delusions and hallucinations are more common in dementia with Lewy bodies (Chiu *et al.*, 2006). Those with Parkinson's dementia tend to have impaired visuo-spatial functioning, hallucinations and paranoia (Emre *et al.*, 2007). It is important to have an understanding of these different types of symptoms because it is often an exacerbation of these that leads to the person requiring long-term care.

Every person with dementia is different. This is not just because of the number of different diseases that are called 'dementia' but also because the part of the brain affected by the disease will influence behaviour. Some people may have more than one type of dementia.

How many different presentations of dementia have you observed in the older people you care for?

Stigma of dementia

There is still stigma attached to mental illness and dementia is often included in this category. Goldsmith (2004) described how a person is treated differently, both consciously and unconsciously, once the diagnosis of dementia is made. People are on the look-out for lapses and personality changes which increases the pressure on the person with the diagnosis of dementia. The person who is supposedly unable to remember is also judged as being unable to understand. It is assumed they have no insight, therefore cannot contribute to decision making about their care or future (Bryden, 2005).

The stigma of dementia is obvious in the rhetoric that is used around dementia. George (2010, p.586) described how we view dementia as a 'battle', how it 'attacks' or 'strikes us down'. The terminology used has a powerful message of war against dementia. He also described how those with dementia experience 'social death' or 'living death' or that carers experience the 'burden of care' (George, 2010, p.586). The headline in *The Independent* declares: 'Britain unprepared for the tsunami of dementia patients' (16 September 2012). In Australia we have the headline in *The Herald Sun*: '"Boomers" crisis over dementia will threaten society's fabric' (23 September 2013).

Ageing is viewed by policy makers as a 'crisis'. Each of these terms reinforces the way we as a society view dementia and ageing. George (2010) contends that the language we use is a very powerful way to provide a negative view of dementia. We should be using language that reflects more than the negative. Think about 'postponement' rather than 'cure' (George 2010, p.587); to remove the stigma of both ageing and dementia and seek the positives from the situation.

Instead of concentrating on the 'burden' of caring, look for the joys, sharing, compassion, forgiveness and reconciliation to be gained from caring. To celebrate the progress in public health that ensures a larger population of older people who provide many strengths, talents and wisdom – George (2010) provides a very powerful message to counteract the stigma of dementia and ageing via semantics.

New ways of thinking about dementia: not only a burden, but also consider the joys, compassion, forgiveness.

Perhaps the greatest stigma of dementia is the societal notion of 'living death' or of having no further functions to fulfil – of being a 'non-person' or having no value. Behuniak (2011, p.71) uses the metaphor of 'zombie' to describe how society seems to view those with dementia – those who are the living dead – constrained by their disease with no sense of self remaining.

She noted that 'zombie' is something that has not only stigma, but is hated and viewed with disgust and fear. This is reinforced by books – there have been a number of publications which characterize Alzheimer's disease and dementia as a living death including books like *Alzheimer's Disease: Coping with a Living Death* (Woods, 1980, cited in Behuniak, 2011). This social construction, she contends, was initiated by the biomedical approach to dementia – the person became a body that needed to be managed rather than a person to be cared for and valued.

Kitwood (1997) noted that the stigma associated with dementia can lead to the person being intimidated, labelled, banished and objectified rather than valued, included and respected. The stigma of dementia had meant that those with dementia and their families are reluctant to discuss their fears and freely make plans for the future. We still, in some settings, find that people don't want to talk about it, especially not to the person who has dementia. Mukerdam and Livingstone (2012) contend that the stigma of dementia from professionals and the public has some very significant impacts for the person and leads to higher carer stress, lower quality of life and worse care planning.

It is also important to think about the associated stigmatization of carers of those with dementia. If, as a society, we view those with dementia a 'zombies' or 'non-persons' or we say that the person is 'no longer the one we knew', how do carers feel about their chosen role? Can carers hold their heads up high when they declare that they work in aged care? If we view those with dementia a 'non-persons' then it is very easy to ignore their emotional and spiritual needs and just concentrate on the basic activities of daily living.

> - How often have you spoken to someone about their memory loss and dementia?
>
> - Is this an easy topic to talk about?
>
> - Have you noticed that people have 'expectations' of someone with dementia?
>
> - We found some families did not want the word 'dementia' mentioned to their loved ones. Why do you think that might be so?

In the spiritual reminiscence research project, we discovered a number of instances of this reluctance to mention that the research was about dementia. In one instance, a participant's son did not mind his mother being in the study as long as we did not mention the word 'dementia'. When seeking consents from relatives to participate in spiritual reminiscence for those with dementia, initially the only consents we received were from people bedridden and in the final stages of Alzheimer's disease – relatives seemed reluctant to admit in earlier stages that their loved one had dementia. Yet, in the spiritual reminiscence groups, people with dementia laughed and made jokes about their lack of memory.

Sometimes family members did not think that the person knew they had dementia and therefore talked about them rather than with them. Yet, in other cases it has been the parent with the dementia who did not want to acknowledge their condition. In one recent group of spiritual reminiscence with people with dementia, the mother had difficulty speaking in the group sessions, and often cried. But then after several weeks, she seemed to be much more at peace. It was after she had died, that her daughter made contact and told Elizabeth (group facilitator) how amazed she had been that during those few weeks, her mother had stopped denying that she had dementia, and came to a state of acceptance of her condition. There had been healing and reconciliation between mother and family.

There sometimes seems to be an assumption that the older person with dementia needs to be protected from reality. This allows very little discussion with the person most affected by dementia – the person who has dementia. It is a little bit like 'don't mention the war!'.

The stigma of dementia impacts directly on those with dementia and their families. Christine Bryden (2012) described how the diagnosis of dementia affected her life. Being just 46 years old, she was not a typical person with dementia. It took her two years before she was able to 'come-out' and declare that she had dementia. During the first period of her disease she felt that she was sliding into depression and living the 'medical model' view of dementia – gradual and exorable decline. Then, two years after the diagnosis, she decided to embrace life – to reject the model of what was supposed to happen and make things happen for herself. She wrote her first book and enrolled in a graduate diploma – not the activities we expect for someone with dementia. She described the stigma she felt as she ceased to be a person and became a person with dementia. In her second book: *Dancing with Dementia* (2005), she recorded the continuing journey into dementia, including re-marriage to Paul. She thus confounded the myth that life does not go on after the diagnosis of dementia.

Stigma impacts directly on the person with dementia and can lead to delay in seeking diagnosis and treatment, loss of self-esteem, reluctance to discuss memory loss with their family and friends, and it influences how society views those with dementia.

Caring for people with dementia: The need to find meaning

An older person entering an aged care facility faces significant losses. There can be loss of: community and friends; possessions; their own home; pets; independence; and privacy. Although relieved of the burden of the day-to-day management of a home, the person may have little or no control over the types of food provided and the people caring for him/her. A person who has valued their independence and privacy is often in the situation of having to rely on others for basic human needs. These losses lead to considerable grief and can include anger, anxiety and fearfulness, mental disorganization and feelings of being overwhelmed. For an older person already managing memory loss, these feelings can create further confusion leading to aggression, paranoia and depression.

The issues around the needs of these people and their care are indeed complex. Post (2006, p.229), writing of our responsibilities in the care of people with dementia says, 'Our task as moral agents is to remind persons with dementia of their continuing self-identity'. An important way of helping people who have dementia to find meaning in the midst of cognitive decline and multiple losses is through engaging in spiritual reminiscence.

Admission to an aged care facility can be the final straw in a number of losses encountered by the older person.

What ways can staff assist new residents in this transition?

What measures do you take to ensure that a person with dementia feels safe, secure and at home?

Importantly, how can people find meaning in the face of these losses and transitions?

Chapter 3

Communication

We have spoken to people with dementia about their hopes and fears, joy and sadness and meaning in life for the last ten years. We have conducted in-depth interviews with over a hundred participants and analyzed hundreds of pages of transcripts of spiritual reminiscence groups. This has led us to believe that the success of spiritual reminiscence is based primarily on excellent communication skills from the group facilitators. In this chapter, we will outline some communication issues and attempt to give some tips for better practice. Although we are concentrating on facilitating spiritual reminiscence groups in this guide, good general communication skills can be applied to any caring situation, residential or community, and with groups or individuals.

These communication skills include: allowing time for responses; watching carefully for non-verbal interactions; skilfully including all in the process; and using thoughtful questioning. Many authors contend that good communication skills from carers are the key to enhancing physical, psychological and spiritual care (Bird, 2002; Goldsmith, 1996; Herman and Williams, 2009; Killick and Allan, 2001; Kitwood, 1993; Naue and Kroll, 2008; and Smith and Buckwalter, 2005). Using spiritual reminiscence is a way to encourage and enhance this communication.

Older people with dementia in residential care rarely speak to each other – it is often that you see groups of chairs around the wall or all facing the television. One study identified that nearly half of all aged care residents never talk to their roommate because of speech or hearing impediments (Kovach and Robinson, 1996). Although we often see groups of people with dementia sitting together, frequently there is little or no communication between them. In fact, even in activity groups the communication goes between the person leading the group and the individual. Yet, in the spiritual reminiscence groups it was often noted how individuals interacted among themselves, enhancing on-going interactions.

People with dementia have difficulty expressing their thoughts. They may have trouble finding the right word, beginning an interaction, concentrating on questions and remarks and ending an interaction. This, however, does not mean that those with dementia have less to say or that what they say is not meaningful. Killick (1997) sat with people in an aged care facility for long periods noting all their spoken communication. These conversations were meaningful and insightful and demonstrated significant ability for expression – among people who often have diminished capacity to find words. Killick noted in the introduction to his book that one of the people with dementia asked: 'who's in charge of spare words?' (1997, p.6).

An account from a pastoral carer working in a dementia specific unit showed that even with advanced dementia, narrative, although fractured, may still be present, if given an opportunity to emerge. The incident involved a woman with dementia sitting alone in a water chair; she had been placed in the room by herself because she kept calling out and disturbed others. The pastoral carer went into the room and simply sat with her quietly for half an hour. It was at that point that the woman said: 'In despair, in the chair…is dull, is horrible, just sitting in this chair… It's not good, could be worse.' This woman, with almost no speech left was able to articulate her distress when someone sat with her for long enough for her to be able to speak it (MacKinlay, 2001).

So, the question arises, 'How can we communicate effectively with people with dementia and promote meaningful interactions that add meaning to daily life?'.

> How can we communicate effectively with people with dementia and promote meaningful interactions that add meaning to daily life?

Frequently communication with those with dementia is superficial, trivial and patronizing. Little emphasis is given to meaningful topics or questions that allow the older person to pose considered responses about things that interest them. This comes about for a number of reasons including lack of time on the part of staff, feeling ill equipped to deal with the responses, and thinking that the person would be unable to communicate adequately to respond.

Kitwood (1997) wrote that the onus is on those without dementia to facilitate the communication, that is, we should not expect the person with dementia to meet our expectations for communication. He provides the analogy of tennis when trying to emphasize this communication. A tennis coach can return any ball hit by a novice – whether or not these shots meet the requirements for a tennis game – the coach can help the novice to keep the rally going – the coach is not aiming to win the game, (Kitwood, 1993). This is a valuable analogy – the role of the carer or facilitator or family member is to keep the communication going – even if it seems the conversation is off track or not meeting our expectations.

> Think back on all your interactions with older people – those with or without dementia. Have you ever asked them what brings meaning, or joy or sadness to their lives?

In his article, 'Dementia and suffering in nursing homes', Michael Bird (2002) described a number of occasions where the suffering was increased for residents as a result of the behaviours of care staff. He illustrated this using three case studies in which residents had significant symptoms leading to difficult behaviours as a result of their dementia. In a number of instances he was surprised that staff believed that the behaviour was done on purpose to annoy and frustrate. Bird suggested that staff seemed to think that: 'many people with advanced dementia wake up each morning thinking to themselves: What clever wheezes can I get up to today to make life hell for the staff?' (Bird, 2002, p.57).

He found that by learning some basic caring skills and identifying the underlying issues to do with the behaviour, staff felt more able to cope with the behaviour. In two cases, staff learned of the background of the person and were able to understand and thus tolerate the behaviour more easily. The third case was that of an older woman with dementia, Joy, who was very combative during personal hygiene activities. She fought and hit out to prevent her clothes being removed and having a shower. The final straw was when she injured two staff members while being showered.

Through interviews with her family, Bird found out that this woman was extremely shy – it was not surprising that she fought against having her clothes removed by those she perceived as strangers. Ironically, a weekend carer showered her with no problems at all, thus reinforcing the message that many symptoms of dementia are exacerbated by interactions with staff. Despite measures to help prevent further injury the damage was done – it was decided to sedate this woman with drastic results. She reacted poorly to the sedatives, became weak and listless and soon died. These case studies demonstrated clearly how reframing of events by staff can have a significant impact on the way the person is treated.

Using spiritual reminiscence with person-centred care is one way to identify and reframe issues.

Person-centred care in communication

The term 'person-centred care' was developed in the early 1990s by Tom Kitwood as part of the Bradford Dementia Research Group. He was frustrated by the biomedical paradigm that suggested that the person with dementia was a set of behaviours to manage until the person died. If you are just managing behaviours then there is no need to interact in a meaningful way. He also contended that much of what happens in older age is socially constructed – that is not happening because of changes as we get older, but more as a response to the way others approach to us – often in response to stigma. Therefore, if we changed our approach to those with dementia then in turn their response would also change.

Person-centred communication recognizes that the person with dementia is respected as a fellow human being who happens to have some special needs. According to Kitwood, we accord an individual the status of a person when we acknowledge his/her:

- unique make-up as an individual

- place in the human group

- needs

- value simply because he is a human being

- rights.

(Kitwood, 1997)

At the heart of a person-centred approach there is an emphasis on a relationship in which there is the capacity for each person to discover something new, creative and nurturing in another person (Goldsmith, 2004). Kitwood describes this as the ability to be present to the person with dementia. It entails letting go of the constant doing involved in dementia care and becoming involved in being with the person (Kitwood, 1997).

Kitwood described ten types of behaviours from carers that undermine person-centred care and reinforce the loss of self and respect for those with dementia. He labelled these a 'malignant social psychology' and included: treachery, disempowerment, infantilization, condemnation, intimidation, stigmatization, banishment and objectification (Kitwood, 1993, p.542). He shifted the emphasis and responsibility for 'difficult behaviours' firmly away from the person with dementia and suggested that these 'difficult behaviours' arise out of a need to exert some kind of independence and autonomy – even in the face of on-going dementia.

He also proposed an opposite set of approaches that enhance and support the sense of individuality and self – again these are carer characteristics and include: recognition, negotiation, play, relaxation, validation, and facilitation. He asked that carers accept and acknowledge creative actions initiated by the person with dementia; and that caregivers are humble enough to accept whatever gift or kindness or support a person with dementia is able to bestow (Kitwood, 1997).

> There are a number of attributes that are required from a carer who is undertaking person-centred care. The person needs to be flexible, open, caring, compassionate and inwardly at ease.
>
> What other behaviours and attributes do you think make up this sort of caregiver?

Principles of good communication

Sometimes when we first met with people who have dementia, and asked them if they would share some of their life story with us, on a one-on-one basis, the person would reply 'But I don't have a story to tell, I'm only an ordinary person' (Trevitt and MacKinlay, 2006, p.79). Yet, when we took time to sit with them and affirm them as people worth listening to, the story would emerge, and gradually with more confidence. When you listen to another person you are acknowledging them as an individual in their own right. Good communication reinforces the notions of person-centred care. People with dementia are in danger of losing their identity because that identity rests on appropriate responses from other people. By not responding, ignoring or belittling the person's story then we are implying that they have no value.

Killick and Allan (2001) described the importance of communication skills when interacting with those with dementia. Issues such as knowledge of the person's life story, listening and not interrupting, taking risks and asking questions we might not feel comfortable about are all important when communicating with this group of older people. John Killick identified some particular communication challenges for people with dementia. Some of these difficulties include:

- getting stuck on one sound and repeating it

- finding the right word

- using words in the wrong way

- using incorrect pronouns (such as him, her, she, it) in confusing ways

- making statements that are repetitive

- speech that has normal words but abnormal structure and thus meaning

- a progressive reduction in speech until it may finally cease altogether.

(Killick and Allen, 2001, p.74)

In our projects, we found that some participants described their difficulty with word-finding. They referred to this in a number of different ways but all were aware of this as a progressive loss due to their increasing dementia. Mabel described the embarrassment she sometimes feels if she cannot find the correct word:

> Mabel: It's hard sometimes to express what you feel, cause you just can't find the right words, and you feel that you sound a bit stupid if you say what you're thinking, you know.
>
> (MacKinlay and Trevitt, 2012, p.205)

Beverly sums this up neatly by saying that 'her brain is shut':

> Beverley: What I worry about? What do I worry about? I can't think of anything special.
>
> Interviewer: You were talking earlier about not finding the right words, does that ever worry you?
>
> Beverley: Oh yes. My brain can be shut.
>
> (MacKinlay and Trevitt, 2012, p.206)

Maureen, in the following excerpt, is responding to some comments made by the facilitator. It is the last week of a six-week group and Maureen is expressing her thanks for the opportunity of the group.

> Maureen: Well I think you have understood, and that helps, what I have. Just that I wanted to be able to express what comes into my brain [it] doesn't come easily to express the way I want it to be expressed.
>
> (MacKinlay and Trevitt, 2012, p.208)

We know that communication is a 'two-way-street' – for someone to communicate, someone has to listen. David Snowden described an amusing incident with an older man with dementia, who had been bedbound for several years and rarely uttered a word. His wife said: 'he doesn't know enough to feel' but in the time with the interviewer, the man did actually speak: 'Imagine his wife's surprise when she suddenly heard her husband's voice from the other room. One of the things he said to the researcher: "I don't talk because no-one listens anymore"' (Snowden, 2001, p.195).

When you listen to another person you are acknowledging them as an individual in their own right. This has been noted in hospital wards where nurses spend far less time interacting with patients with dementia because it is felt that they cannot understand and therefore cannot interact (Ekman *et al.*, 1991). If you receive no response to your story then, after a while, you stop trying to participate or contribute to a conversation.

MacEvoy, Eden and Plant (2014) describe a process of empathetic listening to promote meaningful communication in those with dementia. Through empathetic listening the carer can tune into the experience and needs of those with dementia by: being attentive to different needs; staying calm and relaxed; asking short open-ended questions in the present tense; picking up on emotional cues; being sensitive to pacing issues; searching for the meaning of simple metaphors; and paying close attention to your own emotional response. This involves being very self-aware as well as being able to respond to the person with dementia.

By allowing the person to describe what is going on in their lives, not foreclosing on conversations, and recognizing metaphors, communication can be enhanced and made more meaningful. It can also help to reduce some of the behaviour symptoms that people with dementia can display from frustration. A good example of empathetic communication is between the interviewer and Jennifer. The interviewer feeds back to Jennifer her concerns and gives Jennifer time to respond while demonstrating her on-going interest in the conversation:

Interviewer:	Is there a sense that you have a sense of purpose in your life?
Jennifer:	Oh no, I, oh I don't know what I wanted to say.
Interviewer:	Okay, just take your time.
Jennifer:	I am not remembering things as I used to.
Interviewer:	Right, is that a concern for you?
Jennifer:	Pardon?
Interviewer:	Is that a concern for you?
Jennifer:	Well, I don't seem to be as free as I was. What do you want to know?

(MacKinlay and Trevitt, 2012, p.206)

The following is from the initial interview with Jim. During the interview he spoke about his pleasure in fishing – when asked about any troubles he responded as follows:

Interviewer:	Do you worry about any things now?
Jim:	Yeah. Ah I forget them as soon as I catch them.
Interviewer:	Oh right, yeah.
Jim:	Cause, I'm generally bang, let them go again see? That's all I used to do.
Interviewer:	When you had a worry you took care of it quickly did you?
Jim:	Yeah, I'd just go and seek the best section.

(MacKinlay and Trevitt, 2012, p.211)

Jim's response is a good example of empathetic communication (MacEvoy *et al.*, 2014) and searching for the meaning of 'simple metaphors'. Jim has had a long love of fishing and he responds by talking about how he 'let them go again' and looks for 'the best section' (of the river) when discussing his troubles. He has responded to the question asked – just perhaps not in the way we might expect.

One of the difficulties of communication for those with dementia is the time it takes for them to prepare and verbalize a response. Think about the steps involved in preparing a response to a question for those who are cognitively intact. First you have to be able to hear the question.

Age related hearing loss is one of the most frequent ageing changes in the older population. In Australia, up to 74 per cent of people over the age of 70 years have hearing loss (Access Economics, 2006). Figures are similar in the UK (Allen *et al.*, 2003). Once you have managed to hear the question (often over the din of 'normal noise' in a residential aged care facility), you then need to process the meaning of that question and begin to formulate an answer. When you have decided what you are going to say you need to find the words and verbalize your response hoping that the person has stopped talking long enough to hear your response – or not asked another question.

In recent unpublished research (MacKinlay *et al.*, 2011) we have found that it sometimes takes 5–6 seconds after a question for the person with dementia to be able to respond, far longer than for people without cognitive deficits. It is important to realize that the person may well be able to indicate their wants and needs, given sufficient time and support to await an unhurried reply. The following example demonstrates some of the issues when there is not enough time given for participants to respond. It is interesting to note that another participant (Hetty) recognized that Louise needed more thinking time.

Facilitator:	What do you worry about Louise?
Louise:	Oh I don't really.
Facilitator:	Favourite worries?
Louise:	No I don't.
Facilitator:	What do you think about most of the time?
Louise:	Oh I don't know, I don't know.
Hetty:	She has no time to think.
Facilitator:	No time to think.

(MacKinlay and Trevitt, 2012, p.214)

In the following example the facilitator gave as much time as needed to help Jessica find what she wanted to say. By just affirming that she was still listening the participant was encouraged to keep going – to try to find the right words. The interaction also identifies how frustrating it can be for people with dementia to join in and contribute when words are difficult to find.

Facilitator:	Mmm
Jessica:	I want to do it, but I am slow. And that is the main problem I think, that I am slow at doing these things. I know how to do it, but it doesn't come.

Facilitator:	Mmm hmm
Jessica:	I am slow to get that done, and I keep thinking about it, but it is not coming as quickly as I wanted to, and I am slowly exasperated.
Facilitator:	Mmm.

(MacKinlay and Trevitt, 2012, p.215)

> How many older people with dementia have one or more of these difficulties in communication?
>
> What are some of the tips you have learned over the years to enhance communication and counteract some of these difficulties?

'Elder speak'

The term 'elder speak' has been coined to express the patronizing style of speaking that is sometimes used to older people, it includes raising the tone of voice, speaking down to them as though older people have little ability to understand; this may be used even more in some instances with people who have dementia. Other examples are the use of the plural pronoun (are *we* ready for *our* bath) and inappropriate terms of endearment (Williams *et al.*, 2009). In many respects it is the way we speak to children – it demonstrates disrespect and belittling. Even though a person has dementia they will recognize this lack of respect and respond accordingly. Kitwood (1997, p.46) includes this as one of his aspects of 'malignant social psychology' and describes it as 'infantilism – treating the person with dementia as a child'.

Using elder speak to an older person is not just disrespectful – it has considerable impacts on their self-esteem and sense of worth. Those on the receiving end of elder speak, have their own negative stereotypes reinforced thus eroding self-esteem and the person's evaluation of their capabilities. In a study examining 'elder speak' as a communication style it was found that this predominated and normal adult conversation was infrequent. This study found that there was an increase in behaviour problems and resisting care with both 'elder speak' and silence during care episodes (Herman and Williams, 2009). Other studies have found that elder speak encourages increased dependency especially in residential care settings (Williams *et al.*, 2009).

We noted from our study that it is often easy to slip into these conversation patterns. A few examples of unhelpful communication were:

'Now we're going to have our little discussion group again…'

'You do that all yourself, Joan?'

'She's a clever lady Beryl is?'

These are good examples of paternalistic statements. There was a sense of exasperation in the following interchange:

Facilitator:	Oh yes, just put up with it, do you like anything more to eat, do you normally ask them can I have another piece of toast or something?
Beryl:	Yes.
Facilitator:	You normally do. Is there anything else that makes you fearful or worried?
Beryl:	I don't worry about anything just accept things as they come and deal with them.
Facilitator:	Oh and how do you deal with them?
Beryl:	As they need to be dealt with.
Facilitator:	Yes and how do you do that though, Beryl?
Beryl:	Well the same way as I deal with talking to you.

(MacKinlay and Trevitt, 2006, p.23)

The final statement shows participant insight and a degree of paternalistic questioning and lack of insight by the group facilitator in the communication.

Non-verbal interaction

Non-verbal communication is important in everyday interactions, and according to Burgoon and Bacue 'upwards of 60 per cent of the meaning in any social situation is communicated non-verbally' (2003, p.179). This is also the case for people who have dementia. Being aware of non-verbal cues is an important part of communication with those with dementia especially when it becomes more difficult to speak for them or to express themselves using words. In the groups, people helped each other and used non-verbal interactions to reinforce the relationships in the groups. Hubbard *et al.* (2002) in their study of non-verbal behaviours found that these interactions were very important as part of the social interactions of people with dementia. They found that non-verbal behaviours were used to initiate, enhance and maintain conversations, to amplify interactions, to describe situations they could not find words for or to draw attention quietly to personal needs.

Humour in communication

In the spiritual reminiscence groups there was much laughter as participants laughed at themselves and their situation or recalled amusing past events. Kimble claims that humour may express a 'heroic defiance in the face of life's most crushing and challenging experiences' (Kimble, 2004, p.7). Humour is very important in facing life's adversities. The ability to see humour in even the most dire of events is viewed as an important coping mechanism. This can occur by offering a different way of viewing the adversity – and perhaps leading to laughter which can help to overcome feelings of depression, anxiety or anger (Martin, 2009).

Laughter is also reputed to provide a number of additional physiological benefits. Berk (2010) has summarized a number of these including improved respiration and circulation; decreased stress hormones; increased levels of endorphins; and improved mental functioning. He proposes that 'laughter does offer sedentary elderly folk an alternative' (p.332) and suggests that adding laughter to an exercise program or even replacing the exercise program with laughter is a definite advantage. Kitwood (1993) has identified humour as one of his twelve indicators of personal well-being in moderate or severe dementia. Social interactions of those with dementia are significantly limited – the sharing of laughter can help to enhance the bonds between those with dementia and their family and community.

In the following excerpt Rose makes the group laugh with her humour:

Facilitator: What's the best part of the day, Rose?

Rose: After dinner. I have fallen, after 10 minutes I am off to sleep, and I wake up when it's tea-time.

[Everyone laughs.]

(MacKinlay and Trevitt, 2012, p.114)

The following discussion arose from a question about reading the Bible. It shows a great deal of humour and genuine fun – and identifies how despite older age and dementia – a strong sense of humour prevails. This is also quite a complex interaction between two participants – the facilitator joins in later in the interaction but has not done anything to keep the conversation going.

Ruby: But to me the Bible is very sombre book – don't hear anyone smiling or laughing do you in the Bible – not at all.

Bob: Well, why should it be – I wonder do they laugh when they're not writing Bible stories?

Ruby: I like to hear some fun – very sombre.

Bob: It is – very serious.

Ruby: Yes.

Bob: There's no light heartedness in it at all – it's all serious.

Facilitator: It's serious you're saying.

Bob: Yes very serious…

Facilitator: You don't think it's serious or not – joking funny laughing.

Bob: I think being about God it would have to be – well, it wouldn't have to be serious – no but they made it like that – they haven't recorded any of their happiest days – they're all dismal – you can see them all with long faces like the pictures of them. Can't you Ruby?

Ruby: Yes, and I think it's something that happened in those days perhaps.

Bob: I'm not sure – they must have had a laugh and a giggle I think – oh, they'd have to – but they haven't recorded any of that.

(MacKinlay and Trevitt, 2012, pp.114–15)

It is also good to see how the group picks up on the humour the facilitator uses:

Facilitator: What are you looking forward to Louise?

Louise: Oh, I am too tired [laughs]. Time to get things right, really.

Facilitator: I hope that we will finish this discussion.

                 [Everyone laughs.]

(MacKinlay and Trevitt, 2012, p.115)

Using humour can help older people reframe past events. Even those events surrounding death of loved ones can be reframed by focusing on almost prosaic events that happened in connection with the painful events. Humorous stories are an effective strategy for thinking through negative life events that are intrinsic to being a great age (Matsumoto, 2009). We can see this demonstrated in the group interactions – often laughter was associated with participants talking about either potentially sad events such as their own death, or past sad events.

In the following excerpt we can see how the theme of life and death is discussed with some humour. One of the participants – aged 97 – was frequently bemoaning the fact that she did not have long to live. This became a repeated theme during the 24 week group.

Freda: See I haven't got long to live.

Mavis: Oh, here we go again!

Facilitator: It was bound to come up, wasn't it?

June: Look, tell us when to wring the handkerchiefs.

Freda: No… I've err three years to live.

June: Who told you that?

Facilitator: Is that just because you'll be one hundred in three years? That doesn't mean that's when you have to finish, you can go on to be one hundred and ten.

Mavis: Then you'll be here to annoy us.

Facilitator: That's right. And we'll all be saying, when you're 105 – I thought you said you were going when you were one hundred.

(MacKinlay and Trevitt, 2012, pp.115–16).

Communication about death and dying

As we can see from the section on humour – those with dementia are not afraid to speak about death and dying. As a facilitator you will also need to feel comfortable about these types of topics. When we asked about meaning in life, participants were able to describe the things that they held dear, the precious relationships they had and what made life worthwhile. When we asked them about grief they had experienced and what hopes they had for the future, they were just as frank.

An important distinction that we found between cognitively intact older people, and those with dementia in this study was the relative ease with which more of those with dementia spoke about dying and death. They were more likely to name death as death, not 'passed away'. Grief seemed to be a normal topic among the participants, both in their small groups and individually. Fear of dying was not so marked, while it was a real fear for cognitively intact older people (MacKinlay, 2006).

Dying and death are not often topics raised with people who have dementia. Frequently, families feel uncomfortable in discussing issues of death and dying, both among themselves, and certainly with those who have dementia. It is often said, that the person with dementia will not remember, and it is distressing for them to be told about the death of loved ones, so why mention it in the first place? However, this has not been our experience. In two of the groups, participants died during the project, between one week's session and the next. All participants gained comfort from discussing the interactions and pleasure they had shared with the participant who had died. The following examples identify how comfortable many of the participants were in talking about death:

Carol: Well, you see, a lot of people are you know, frightened, or what else is the word, of dying, but we all have to go, so I just [pause].

Rodney: A long time looking forward to the time when the Lord calls me.

   I know I am going to die; everybody will die, where the end will be.

   That I'll be ready when the Lord calls me, I should be satisfied, be able to say that the Lord has forgiven me, all off in debt.

Maureen: Well, I look forward to going to heaven, that's all I can say. I live from day to day, and that is about all I can say. I go to bed at night, I ask the Lord to look after me, I get up in the morning, I do the same, and that's all I can do.

Bronwyn: I look forward to the family being so close to me, and I know that I am prepared everything has been arranged. And I thank the Lord for my family… I would like to say how happy I am that I live here and I can, if there was anything I could do to help anybody, anyone less fortunate than I, um I'd try to.

(MacKinlay and Trevitt, 2012, pp.172–3)

If these people who have dementia can and do speak of dying and death, should those who do not have dementia also learn to speak of these topics? What is now needed are care providers who can meet people with dementia on their terms, and freely discuss topics that are on the minds and in the hearts of these people.

Most participants in this study described grief as being part of life. When asked about their experiences of grief, for example: Claire gave a response typical of others in the study, saying:

Oh, when relations, you know, mother and father and husband and so forth, when they passed away, but they are the normal griefs and everyone has them. Nothing spectacular though.

(MacKinlay and Trevitt, 2012, p.173)

How comfortable do you feel when discussing grief, loss and death with older people? Has this been something that you would discuss?

The importance of effective communication in facilitating a spiritual reminiscence group

The success of a spiritual reminiscence group is largely based on the skills of the facilitator. Communication with those with dementia can be challenging but the facilitator ensures that all participants are able to connect fully and contribute within the group. A facilitator does not lead or direct but rather guides, supports and affirms the work of the group. The role of the facilitator is to tune in to the needs of the group and identify ways to bring out the best from each member of the group. It is important that the facilitator:

- is able to demonstrate a genuine interest in being with these people

- gives time for the group members to share (and this may mean quite a long time)

- is comfortable sitting in silence with the group members

- appropriately interprets body language

- is respectful of each person's contribution

- encourages quieter group members to contribute.

The skill of the facilitator is to draw the participants into deeper sharing, at the same time maintaining a level of comfort within the group. This group time is in effect, sacred time.

The group time is for the group members to share, not for entertainment by the facilitator. The skill of the facilitator is to draw the participants into deeper sharing, at the same time maintaining a level of comfort within the group.

The facilitator needs to always be listening to the participants and being ready, if needed, to reflect back to the participants and clarify issues. Even so, simply paraphrasing may be confusing for the participants who have difficulty with language. The challenge is to reflect back simply, while not patronizing the speakers.

Be guided by the needs of the participants

Although there is a specific theme with suggested topics for reflection and discussion allocated to each week's meeting, if there are issues that arise, be flexible and spend time on these – do not feel that you must rush through to 'cover' all the questions. One example of participant issues recorded in various of the weekly sessions was the need to address issues of grief.

The facilitator needs to be very comfortable with the notion of personhood and be able to identify the behaviours that lead to malignant social psychology. In addition, she/he needs to have a good understanding of the elements of behaviour that encourage person-centred care and also the guidelines for managing reminiscence activities. Participants in the study seemed quite sensitive to the comfort levels of the facilitator and this was related to how much interaction occurred in the particular group session.

The facilitator also needs to be aware of their own spirituality to be comfortable with the types of questions asked in spiritual reminiscence. One group facilitator in the study, with support of the researchers, decided not to continue facilitating a group as, although she felt this was important work, she did not feel comfortable speaking about spirituality with others.

'What' questions are more likely to elicit responses from the participants. The word 'what' invites a response rather than a 'yes' or 'no' answer.

The skills used in small groups are those used by the helping professions, first, active listening, and being really present with the participants. Effective facilitation of group participation includes using appropriate and open ended questions and then allowing space and silence while the individual reflects. It includes the use of paraphrasing, unconditional acceptance and the skills of focusing and summarizing. But be careful in using paraphrasing, as the person with dementia may be trying to respond to the previous statement or question, and may become more confused when a second statement worded slightly differently is spoken.

Facilitators of spiritual reminiscence groups benefit from experiencing the process themselves, prior to facilitating spiritual reminiscence with other people.

It is important that small group facilitators first experience the process of spiritual reminiscence; it is only by engaging in spiritual reminiscence that individuals will come to an appreciation of the value of the process. In spiritual reminiscence, it is best to focus on the meaning of events and experiences in the lives of the participants rather than simply on the description of the events remembered. This moves the conversation to a deeper level and enables review of life-meaning. Spiritual reminiscence is one of the spiritual tasks of ageing, and as such is an important component of the life journey; it is so much more than simply an activity.

An essential beginning for group work is respect by the group facilitator for the group members and a willingness to meet them where they are in their life journeys.

Communication strategies to enhance spiritual reminiscence

Communication with those with dementia can be challenging at times. Work by Bird (2002) and Kitwood (1997) to name a few, clearly identifies that the onus is on those without dementia to meet the communication needs of those with dementia – not the other way around. There are many authors who have collated 'tips' for communicating with those with dementia. The following tips come from our experiences of spiritual reminiscence over the last ten years.

- Be aware of your own spirituality and be prepared to discuss issues of meaning in life, joy, sadness, loss, grief and death.

- Avoid patronizing conversations and 'elder speak'.

- Introduce simple topics based on the weekly themes.

- Give each participant time to prepare and verbalize a response.

- Demonstrate a caring supportive attitude when waiting for a response.

- Use person-centred communication and recognize the unique contribution that everyone can make.

- Be aware that the use of metaphors is a powerful way that those with dementia can make their meaning clear.

- Assist those with hearing difficulties by sitting them close to the facilitator and helping them to join in with the group.

- Recognize that not all people with dementia will be able to contribute in a group at the start, but given patience and opportunity may well be able to contribute later.

- Identify those people for whom one-on-one spiritual reminiscence work may be the most effective way to proceed.

- Use empathy to help to clarify meaning for the person.

- Be aware and supportive of non-verbal interactions.

- Be flexible and meet the person where they are at in their spiritual needs.

- Do not be afraid of silence while the person with dementia forms a response to the topic.

> We have provided a number of strategies for communication. What are some of the strategies you have used over the years?

Chapter 4

Reminiscence work

Story and narrative gerontology

Reminiscence has been defined by a number of people and it is essentially the process of recalling the past (de Medeiros, 2014). This may consist of a single memory or a series of collected memories (Gibson, 1998, 2004). Reminiscence work was presented first in the early sixties by Robert Butler as life review (Butler, 1995). He saw this life review as being part of a normal review process brought about by the realization of approaching death. A life review may occur as nostalgia, mild expressions of regret and storytelling. In some cases the regrets can generate anxiety, depression and despair. On the other hand, the life review may assist the story teller in coming to appreciate their life-meaning and purpose.

In many cases life review gives people an opportunity to reflect on their accomplishments, gives an opportunity to right old wrongs, reconcile with enemies and become ready to die (Butler, 1995). Butler wrote that this is not always encouraged. Older people have been told that this type of nostalgia is 'living in the past and a pre-occupation with self' (Butler, 1995, p.xvii). He counters this attitude with the proposition that life review should be considered as part of a natural healing process. More recently, there has been an increase in the notions of maintaining and constructing family, local and oral history. Reminiscence has come to be seen as a positive rather than a negative activity and has been recognized as a valuable activity with educational, recreational, social and therapeutic benefits (Gibson, 1998, 2004).

> If you were going to tell your life story what experiences would you include?
>
> Reflect on why you have chosen those experiences.

Telling of a life story has often been seen in terms of simply reminiscing. Webster and Haight (2002) differentiate between the concepts of life review and reminiscence. They propose that reminiscence has little structure and may jump from event to event as memories are triggered. Life review, on the other hand is more of a sequential and structured telling of a life story. Life review tends to be more detailed. They contend that reminiscence is a small part of the life review. They are both ways of recalling the past.

With a growing literature available on reminiscence some debate has focused on whether reminiscence is best used to assist older people to enjoy times of positive remembering, and whether it may be inadvisable to encourage the reminiscence of negative aspects of earlier life. If we consider Erikson's stages (Erikson, Erikson and Kivnick, 1986) of psychosocial development, it seems pertinent to include all life experiences. The struggle that occurs in the final stage of life development between integrity and despair, may enable the person to review and reframe earlier life experiences. In fact the remembering and reprocessing of earlier negative memories may enable the person to move towards ego-integrity in later life and feel a sense of peace.

The value of sharing past disturbing or negative experiences

To deny the existence of disturbing or negative memories may move the person towards a blockage of psychosocial and spiritual growth in later life.

Taking this perspective, Coleman investigated the task of reconciliation for older people, noting that normally reminiscence is rewarding for both the speaker and the listener, however, this is obviously not so with painful memories (Coleman, 1999). Coleman notes that the healing and reconciling focus of life review has been neglected, despite Butler's early work in the 1960s.

In a study of older people and their war memories (WWII) Coleman noted that where disturbing memories remained un-integrated it was necessary to make the original experience explicit 'by categorising and understanding it, for it to lose its power to haunt us' (Coleman, 1999, p.136). He describes the characteristics of a 'successful' story as being one that bears on the subject of reconciliation or harmony between the past, present and future.

A 'successful' story is one that bears on the subject of reconciliation or harmony between the past, present and future.

Faith Gibson (2004) has written extensively on the value and the practicalities of using reminiscence for older people. During the last 30 years she has practised all aspects of life story and reminiscence to improve quality of life for many older people. She contends that reminiscence:

- encourages a sense of coherence and continuity

- encourages sociability and opens up new relationships

- confirms personal identity and encourages feelings of self-worth

- assists the process of life review

- changes the nature of the caring relationships and contributes to staff development

- aids assessment of present functioning and informs managed care plans

- helps to transmit knowledge, values and wisdom and to bear witness.

(Gibson, 2004)

It is interesting to note that reminiscence can help staff as well as the older person. In the spiritual reminiscence project we found that reminiscence certainly encouraged and assisted relationship building in the aged care facility. The stories from the reminiscence also enhanced the caring relationships between carer and resident as each gained a deeper understanding of the other. Situations such as Bird (2002) described could be lessened with this deeper understanding (see Chapter 3). Learning to know the resident as a person changes the way we see them and the ways we may provide care. The stories help to give the residents that sense of identity in the eyes of carers that Bird (2002) has said is so important. We can then become partners in care.

Reminiscence work with people with dementia

Gibson (2004) identifies some general guidelines for working with people with dementia when undertaking reminiscence work. These guidelines are just as important when forming spiritual reminiscence groups. These guidelines include:

- Provide consistency of approach and take time to establish trust.

- Stress mutual pleasure and enjoyment.

- Slow down and make time for responses to be made and conveyed.

- Take the initiative in reaching out and in making and sustaining contact.

- Read and respond to changes to mood, energy and interest.

- Match triggers (if used) to the known life experience and past interests of the person.

- Stress non-verbal activities.

- Believe rather than disbelieve the story being told – suspend judgment.

- Try to decode symbolic conversation. (Some people may use words that are not immediately obvious in their meaning, but symbolize something to the speaker.)

- Avoid challenging the truthfulness of the story.

- Respond to the emotional content of what is being said.

- Be prepared to enter the world of the person with dementia and to validate his or her experience.

- Be flexible and prepared to vary your approach.

- Use reminiscence in its own right and as a passport to creative artistic activities.

- Always seek consent and convey respect.

(Gibson, 2004, p.247)

Obstacles to reminiscence

There are obstacles to story telling – first, having no one to listen; in aged care facilities busyness of staff seems to deter residents from sharing. Coleman (1999) in a study of older people in a hospital found that 30 per cent would like to speak about their life story but felt that they had no one willing to listen.

At initial individual interviews in a recent study of older people with dementia in spiritual reminiscence groups, a number of participants thought they had nothing to contribute to any discussion. They declared that theirs was an 'ordinary life' and thus not worth speaking about (Trevitt and MacKinlay, 2006). It is interesting to speculate about why a person may have come to this opinion about the value of their story.

Some older residents seem to have forgotten their story, perhaps through the lack of opportunities for sharing, while others may not see connection between the past and now, and still others have traumatic experiences they wish to shut out of consciousness.

In those older people with dementia an important reason for saying they had nothing to tell was because no one had sat down with them and appeared interested in listening to their stories. We certainly found this to be so as many of these older people did share their stories with us.

The skills adopted by the facilitator can also be an obstacle to reminiscence. We have already discussed the issue of silence and how this may impact on an interaction. When leading a reminiscence group, the facilitator needs to be aware of and allow silence so the participants can take their time to complete their conversations. Complex questions with too many choices can also impede reminiscence, as can answering for the person.

> Think about your own life story from a purely reminiscent perspective.
> How might this change as you age?

Chapter 5

Spiritual reminiscence

Spiritual reminiscence is a way of telling a life story with an emphasis on what gives meaning to life, what has given joy or brought sadness. The process of spiritual reminiscence may identify things that caused anger, guilt or regret. Exploring some of these issues in older age may help people to reframe some of these events and come to a new understanding of the meaning and purpose of their lives.

Spiritual reminiscence assists participants to find meaning in life in the present, and develop strategies to accept changes of later life, including losses of significant relationships, and increasing disability. It offers people with dementia the chance to talk about their fears, hopes and what they look forward to as they come to the end of their life. For those who hold a faith perspective of life, spiritual reminiscence can assist them to grow spiritually, through reflecting on the place of God and the faith community in the life journey. Outcomes of spiritual reminiscence work include facilitating transcendence and finding hope in the face of increasing vulnerability.

Spiritual reminiscence offers people with dementia the chance to talk about their fears, hopes and what they look forward to as they come to the end of their life.

The recently completed research project (MacKinlay and Trevitt, 2012) identified that long-term participation in a spiritual reminiscence group had statistically significant effects in residents in aged care who have dementia. One hundred and thirteen older adults in aged care facilities, all of whom had dementia, participated. They were allocated to spiritual reminiscence groups to participate in small group work, meeting weekly over a period of either six weeks or six months.

In these small groups, a facilitator would lead a discussion based on spiritual reminiscence. New relationships were developed among group members that improved the experience and quality of life for these people in aged care. Some groups decided to keep meeting after the completion of the project.

Different settings and who does spiritual reminiscence benefit?

Spiritual reminiscence is of value to anyone, whether they have dementia or not. In one sense, it is part of a naturally occurring process that happens for many people as they grow older. The questions usually start to arise in mid life, when the person starts to think about their purpose and meaning in life.

Questions such as:
- *Why am I here?*
- *What is my purpose in life?*
- *Have I been living a purpose filled life?*
are common.

As people become aware of their own mortality, the urgency of these questions tends to grow, for many, but not all.

Reminiscence itself is often enjoyable and has become very popular in ageing and aged care circles in recent decades. Spiritual reminiscence takes it to another level. It provides a depth for exploring these questions. It is valuable in helping people to make sense of their lives. It is part of the continuing growth and development of the spiritual dimension in later life, in both religious and secular contexts.

Spiritual reminiscence is of value for both individuals and for use in small groups. This guide focuses on the benefits and ways of facilitating spiritual reminiscence among people who have dementia. The process of spiritual reminiscence as presented in this learning guide is based on the Model of Spiritual Tasks and Process of Ageing, developed by Elizabeth MacKinlay through research (MacKinlay, 2001, 2006). See Chapter 1 of this guide for a description of the model.

Spiritual reminiscence is of value to individuals and to people in small groups.

Although through this guide we discuss working in small spiritual reminiscence groups, there are a number of pros and cons for this. As we mentioned in the communication chapter (Chapter 3), there are occasions when working one-on-one may be of more benefit to the individual. The benefits of working one-on-one include:

- The person may feel more comfortable sharing with only one other person.
- It may be easier to share more difficult topics and memories that have been distressing for the person.
- Some people don't like to speak in groups.

There are, however, many benefits to working in small groups. These include:

- the bonding experience as people in the group realize that they have experienced similar life events
- participants in small groups were comfortable in sharing deep and sometimes difficult memories
- often participants in the group would be supportive of the person sharing difficult life events
- memories of special life experiences can be shared and celebrated together
- being in a small group over time helped the group members to become friends with others in the group.

All our work has been done with people in residential aged care as it proved difficult to set up groups in community settings for the study and trial of the programs. However, spiritual reminiscence has been successfully used in community settings as well. In fact, it would benefit those who have early onset dementia or Alzheimer's disease to take part in spiritual reminiscence. Elizabeth worked with Christine Bryden (Bryden, 2012, Bryden and MacKinlay, 2002) after she was diagnosed with dementia in the mid 1990s in an individual spiritual reminiscence process that set in motion the original ideas for researching this process and setting up this program.

The importance of community and mutual support is highlighted in the words of Christine Bryden as she has experienced the need for others in living with dementia:

> As I travel towards the dissolution of myself, my personality, my very 'essence', my relationship with God needs increasing support from you, my other in the body of Christ. Don't abandon me at any stage, for the Holy Spirit connects us. It links our souls, our spirits – not our minds or brains. I need you to minister to me, to sing with me, pray with me, to be my memory for me. (Bryden and MacKinlay, 2002, p.74)

It is in this context of connecting with others that we have found small group work in spiritual reminiscence to be particularly effective.

Chapter 6

The process of small group spiritual reminiscence

Spiritual reminiscence is a process of engaging with life – meaning: not an activity.

The facilitator, reminiscence and group size

The role and skills required of the facilitator were discussed in Chapter 3.

Although a facilitator can work effectively with up to six participants this is dependent on the participants. If the group has more than six participants, it will not be possible for all to be engaged in the process. If any participants have hearing deficits, diminished ability to speak or diminished concentration span, the groups should be smaller.

Larger groups often result in some participants being left out and not having the opportunity to become engaged in the process. Concentration span can be reduced in those who have greater cognitive deficits and it works best to assign participants who have similar levels of communication ability to the same group.

We have found that over longer-term groups, the participants' abilities to communicate within the groups does increase and it has been surprising to follow through the transcripts of sessions for the six month groups and see how the people have increasingly interacted with each other.

Depending on the topic chosen for the day, the group session may vary in length from 30 minutes to an hour. We have also found in sessions that explore the participants' faith and relationship with God, that it is important for the group facilitator to be comfortable in talking about issues of faith; if the facilitator is uncomfortable, this will readily be communicated to the participants, especially if the group members have dementia.

This box of questions was posed during Chapter 1 of this guide. Complete these again – have any of your responses changed as a result of your reading so far?

Speaking to others about spirituality

Before we go any further, it will be helpful to explore your spiritual core.

Think about and answer the following:

- What gives you most meaning in your life?

- Looking back over your life so far:

    » What has made you feel happy or sad?

    » What has brought you joy?

    » Do you have any regrets?

    » Do you have any fears for the future?

- Do you have any religious or spiritual practices that are important to you?

- What or who is most important in your life?

How do you feel about providing spiritual care for people from different cultures and faiths and those who may or may not have a religious faith?

The meeting place

It is helpful to have a designated meeting place so that participants become comfortable with that environment. It can take quite a bit of negotiation to find the best time and place to hold the weekly sessions. Aged care facilities can sometimes be very noisy and it is difficult for residents to concentrate and to hear the other group members speaking. One of the groups we facilitated occurred during the facility renovations – this added greatly to the challenge of engaging the participants! Do make sure that participants with hearing deficits have their hearing aids on and working. Some facilitators have found that positioning hard of hearing residents near to them helps to encourage understanding and contribution. Make sure that participants have their glasses clean and on.

Meeting timing

The timing of the group meeting is important. It needs to be at a time when there are not other activities taking place in the facility. The time chosen should be when the participants are not too tired to interact. Sometimes juggling times with excursions, music and other activities is difficult. We have also found that trying to keep the meeting time similar each week assists with gathering people for the group. In fact in one aged care facility the members of the longer groups seemed to know when the meeting was due to be held and voluntarily came to the meeting place each week in anticipation of the spiritual reminiscence activity. This was not a common occurrence for other activities.

A six week cycle of questions for the spiritual reminiscence program

We have found that repetition of certain topics over 24 weeks with groups gives the greatest responses. As each group progresses, trust develops between the participants, and with each repetition of topics more information is offered, and the sharing increases. Group topics for spiritual reminiscence are based on MacKinlay's Spiritual Tasks and Process of Ageing Model (2001) and used in a Linkage Grant project 2002–2005.

It seems to work best when one topic is introduced at a time, and all participants are given an opportunity to contribute in turn, before introducing another topic. In some cases of people with greater communication difficulties, we noticed they would answer an earlier question later in the session. So it is important to really listen to the participants' responses.

A series of six themes of broad topics can be used to facilitate the process of spiritual reminiscence over six weekly group sessions. The choice of these themes and topics was based on the research (MacKinlay, 2001, 2006) which examined where older people found meaning in their lives. This is not a Q&A session, but rather, an invitation to engage in story listening and story telling. The broad topics below are suggested outlines for each weekly session. Included is some dialogue that was audio-recorded and transcribed from the research study of reminiscence groups (MacKinlay and Trevitt, 2005, 2012). The responses from many of the participants were rich and full of meaning. The spiritual reminiscence groups that were held for 24 weeks used these same questions over four six-week cycles.

Our research has shown that changes in behaviour in aspects of interaction have increased over time during these 24 week programs. Residents remembered their interactions from the previous times they have responded to these topics – seeming to contradict the notions that they 'cannot remember recent events'. Often memory of previous events was related to the meaning these events held for participants.

Table 6.1 The main weekly themes

Week	Main theme
Week 1	Life-meaning
Week 2	Relationships, isolation and connecting
Week 3	Hopes, fears and worries
Week 4	Growing older and transcendence
Week 5	Spiritual and religious beliefs
Week 6	Spiritual and religious practices

MacKinlay and Trevitt, 2012, p.62

In the following interchanges there are examples of responses to the main topics used in spiritual reminiscence.

All participants have been allocated pseudonyms. When reading these responses, keep in mind that all the participants in the original studies had dementia and were unable to live independently.

In many cases participants interacted with each other rather than through the facilitator. This was more likely to occur in the longer running groups, as they got to know each other better. The observational journals note that participants assisted and responded to each other by touch and presence, when deep or difficult things were shared.

Preparation for the spiritual reminiscence sessions

Preparation by the facilitator for each of the group meetings is important. Perhaps a time of quiet reflection or prayer, of stillness, relaxation or meditation in readiness to be able to be present to the group members, will be of value for both the facilitator and the participants.

People who have dementia often seem to be very sensitive to the mood and anxiety levels of the facilitator. If you have been very busy, or have something else on your mind immediately prior to the session, try to let go of that for the duration of the session.

Knowing something about each of the participants facilitates the beginning of the group sessions, but as facilitator, you will get to know the group members well over the course of the sessions. Knowing the themes for each week ahead of time will allow you to gather any materials that might be of significance to participants, such as photos, scrap books, music, flowers or whatever fits with the participant interests and needs.

Celebrate special occasions: Birthdays, anniversaries or other special markers of life journey.

Use imagination and creativity.

It is important to be aware of group members' understandings of the spiritual dimension and religion, if it is relevant. Some small groups had a combination of people who held a religious faith and those who did not, and these groups still functioned well.

Remember these small group sessions do not focus on what the participants can remember, but the meaning of events and feelings of what is important to them.

The process of spiritual reminiscence has a very different focus from the usual activity of an aged care facility, where activity is emphasized; here *reflection* and *being* are emphasized. The facilitator is present to encourage and facilitate the conversation, not to lead it and certainly not to control the group session. In this process the people with dementia over a period of time are empowered to initiate conversation and to respond to each other in the group, within their capabilities. This time is their time, even though the participants may need support with communication (see Chapter 3 for details on skill development).

It is also important to mention that what is shared each session in the group setting stays within the group and you do not discuss it with other people. At the same time, it may be helpful to let other staff know the main theme that is the focus of each week (without divulging anything confidential), in case participants raise issues related to this theme after the group session. In some care settings there may be a book where the theme of the week can be recorded.

Confidentiality: What is said in the group stays in the group.

In these sessions we have found examples of wisdom, if we understand wisdom as the ability to live with increased uncertainty and ambiguity, 'a deepening search for meaning in life, including an awareness of the paradoxical and contradictory nature of reality' (MacKinlay, 2001, p.153). Meaning is constructed through story and Randall and Kenyon (2004) have highlighted the importance of catching 'storying moments' (Kenyon, 2003, p.31) which can be used to further explore and to affirm the story teller. We often focus so much on memory loss that we fail to see that the present moment is the only reality, for any of us.

The story listener calls forth the words of the story teller (Kenyon, 2003, p.31). This is privileged work.

It is in the community holding the story of the person with dementia with love and respect that affirms and upholds the person who is at the centre of care (for further discussion see MacKinlay and Trevitt, 2012, p.118).

Prior to the spiritual reminiscence session:

- *Find out about the backgrounds of people in your group, as appropriate.*
- *Prepare for the group session – gather any memory prompts, or information.*
- *Ensure the meeting place is ready.*
- *Ensure that others in the facility know that you are running the group and when it is on.*
- *Ensure that support is available if any group members need to talk further with a chaplain or counsellor about any issues that can't be handled adequately in the group.*

Part 2

The weekly sessions of spiritual reminiscence

Guidelines for facilitating the weekly sessions

Part 2 of the learning guide focuses on preparation for and facilitation of the weekly sessions. Numbers of examples from our original research project are included, to give examples of how your participants might respond to the various themes and topics in the program.

Good preparation is vital for effective group work. These guidelines apply to each session, while there is a specific theme for each week with its own special preparation. These sessions are part of the holistic program to support and affirm the well-being of people with dementia. It is therefore important to:

- *Remember to chart the session*: It is important that the session is in the weekly facility program so all staff can be aware of it and incorporate it into the daily plans for the participants. This will ensure that conflicts of appointments are avoided.

- *Chart the theme used*: It is also important to list the theme for the week, so that others may be aware if topics from the sessions are raised at other times.

- *Note who came*: It is helpful to keep a list of attendance at the sessions, and it may be that this is charted in the individual's notes.

An information sheet (Appendix 2) for families and friends of potential participants in spiritual reminiscence groups is to be found on page 103. This is able to be either copied or adapted to meet the needs of each group. (Both appendices at the end of the book can be photocopied.)

Remember: In each group session, the focus is on meaning, emotions and spirituality, not on facts and cognition.

Tips for preparing for the group sessions

Be guided by the needs of the participants in the group, though there are some things you can prepare to help to trigger memories and responses to the weekly topics. Please keep in mind that none of these are hard-and-fast rules – but guidelines you may be able to use.

A set of cards with large print that names the theme for each week's session can be useful. Use these to show the theme for the week to the participants, perhaps placing the card on a central table (if one is used). Or alternatively, give each participant a copy of the main themes for discussion and sharing.

Think about what you might use as resources for each of the sessions. Sometimes gentle relaxation exercises, guided by the facilitator can be used. Music at the start can help the group members to relax. Be guided by group members in what works for them.

Think about the shape of the session: how will you engage the participants' interest? Some questions to ask yourself prior to each session are:

- How will I gain participant interest as the start of the session?

- How will the process of the session unfold?

- How will I bring the session to an effective close?

Some of the weekly themes lend themselves to particular resources. Perhaps a candle, or flowers, or plants, and any particular article that might be meaningful to the participants. Or use photos, craft articles, paintings. In two recent groups that Elizabeth facilitated, one of the participants was an artist. Other members of the group enjoyed seeing paintings done by someone in their own group, and hearing the stories of the paintings. Such examples can be woven into the weekly themes, for example: meaningful activities.

These sessions are part of the holistic program to support and affirm the well-being of people with dementia.

Always accord respect and dignity to each group member, for example, call them by name, avoid using 'elder speak' or using terms such as 'sweetie'.

Facilitator self-care

There may be events in the life of the facilitator that are raised while facilitating these group sessions. For example, perhaps the facilitator has not worked through an experience of grief from their earlier life. This experience may need support to assist the facilitator to effectively deal with the past grief and lay that to rest.

Doing that will free the facilitator to be more fully present to the group members as they deal with their own matters of grief. Involvement in the group where other personal stories of the participants might raise unresolved matters for the facilitator as well and may need to be dealt with.

The facilitator may also be tired and have other things on her mind that make it hard to give of her/himself to the group members.

Having someone on staff that you can share with is valuable. A few staff may form a peer support group and decide to meet together on a regular basis to share the challenging things that they have experienced in the group process, or just when they are not sure how to handle a particular matter. A mentor may provide a valuable listening service for the facilitator.

In some instances, the support may need to be from others engaged in similar work, but in different settings. As in any of these situations, the confidentiality of the group must be observed; however, it is possible to discuss matters of principle without breaching confidentiality. Further, it is good practice not to take work situations home.

If particular personal matters are raised that can't be resolved in a peer group, back-up from a qualified chaplain or counsellor will be of value.

Setting up such structures, both informally and formally in care situations leads to better practice, as the staff are able to talk through issues when they first arise and will feel empowered to work more effectively with those in their care.

Chapter 7

Week 1
Life-meaning

This first week is an important time for settling in and getting to know each other in the group.

Remember what you have learned from the communication chapter (Chapter 3) in this guide – you may want to revise that section before you begin work as a facilitator.

Revise and prepare for the session using the guidelines for Part 2.

Beginning the first group session – tips for the facilitator

Introduction to group members:

Do all the people coming to this first session already know each other?

1. *It is helpful to introduce them to each other.*

2. *Call group members by name.*

3. *Invite them each to share something that they would like others in the group to know about them.*

4. *Be careful not to put pressure on them at this time.*

5. *Connect with the group members, use body language, to invite engagement.*

6. *Explain what the group sessions are about, sufficient for the group members to know why they are there.*

7. *Give time for them to connect with you.*

Week one deliberately begins with the focus on meaning. It provides a good means of introduction to the members, and there can be no sense of failure in responses to the broad topics suggested to guide discussion and responses. Each person's story and where they find meaning is unique, and cannot be judged by anyone else. Sometimes when we interviewed people with dementia individually prior to starting, they would say that they didn't have a story to tell. With encouragement, the story emerged. Then later nearly every one of them did have contributions to make to the group.

This week is about where the participants in the new group find meaning in their lives.

We all have a story to tell but we may never have had the chance to tell our story to another person. People who have dementia still have a story to share.

The first week begins with a very significant topic:

> What gives greatest meaning to your life now?

Experience shows us that many older people with dementia have little difficulty either understanding or answering this question. Some facilitators have tried asking questions like 'What gets you up every morning?' to elicit responses but often these are taken quite literally and participants talk about breakfast, or the nurse who helps them get out of bed! For the person with dementia, they are more likely to respond to the question about meaning than to a question that calls for a factual answer. In other words, these are not so much questions as the starting point for exploration of the important things in the person's life.

People with dementia find it easier to respond to topics about meaning and emotions than to factual questions.

A suggested introduction to Week 1

Each person has a unique life story. In this group we want to give you the opportunity to share some of the important parts of your life journey.

This is your group and your time.

There are times in life that are important and have shaped our lives, some of these have brought joy through the various experiences of life.

Some experiences have been sad. You might like to share some of these, please feel free to share any or none of these, just as you feel comfortable.

Allow time for the group to take this in before continuing.

Depending on the cognitive levels of the group members, the following explanation about the rest of the weekly themes may be included in the introduction or omitted:

These sessions are about exploring your life stories and the important things in them. They will focus on a single theme each week.

The themes are:

- meaning in life

- relationships and connecting

- hopes, fears and worries

- what's it like growing older

- where do you find deepest meaning – spirituality and/or religion

- your spiritual or religious practices: worship, sacred texts, prayer, study, meditation, art, music.

(MacKinlay and Trevitt, 2012; MacKinlay, 2001, 2006)

This first week we will begin with exploring and sharing about where each of you find meaning or purpose in life.

A card with the main themes for each week may be placed on a small table or somewhere that the participants can see it. (Large print and colourful.)

It can be referred to during the session to help bring participants back onto the theme.

Topics for week 1

1. What gives greatest meaning to your life now?

Some may respond to use of the word 'purpose' rather than meaning. And you may follow up with further entry points to exploring meaning like:

- What is most important in your life?

- What keeps you going?

- Is life worth living?

- If life is worth living – why is it worth living? If not, then you might like to ask – why do you feel life is not worth living?

2. Looking back over your life:

- What do you remember with joy?

- What do you remember with sadness?

- What gives greatest meaning to your life now?

We provided examples below of what participants spoke of as most important to them, and what brought meaning. These are the actual words of the people who have dementia:

Claire:	Oh well I suppose getting married and having my daughter, things like, things that normally happen.
Daphne:	Just thinking about the future, and the future for me, is to go and, uh, at one time, when he is ready, uh, put me into, um, a place that he has prepared for me.
Facilitator:	Yes.
Daphne:	And this is really my whole heart, the other is just struggling along, as you will find most of us are.
	We struggle along, some better than others, and my hearing is quite good, my sight is awful, I can hardly see anything, and my walking is awful, I can't do very much, but I still manage to go out on the bus, and that affords some relief, some different atmosphere, so to speak, and as long as I get that to walk here, in here, that sort of, hasn't got wheels on it, you will see, just slides along, so it's not suitable to take outside, but as long as I can get to the bus stop which is just across the road…
Daphne:	So I manage very well, but um, when you say *what is the greatest thing,*[1] *in a way there is not anything on earth because I just think that my journey is almost to the end, and I am hoping it is,* uh, not, not, I was depressed last week, not very often I am, but what with the kitchen and everything else all being out of order, and everybody being at their wit's end, and not knowing what what's where, and it's, um, I do feel, a lot better this week, and I have got back to normal again now.

The participant in the exchange above came back to the original question (of the good things in life) some time later, and reflected on her life journey. She seemed to be looking to life after death in the comment above, in italics (MacKinlay and Trevitt, 2012, p.97).

You will notice that relationship is commonly where these people with dementia find meaning.

Just as it is for any other people.

---

[1]   Daphne was responding to an earlier question. It is not uncommon for people with cognitive disabilities to take some time to start to respond to a question. In fact it was only in looking back at the transcripts that we could sometimes see that they were responding appropriately, but to an earlier topic, well passed by in the conversation.

Spiritual reminiscence can be done one-on-one or in small groups:

Where you see 'Interviewer' it means this example is from a one-on-one session.

Where you see 'Facilitator' this is from a small group session.

In the next example, you can read the responses of participants when asked about joy in their lives; this taps into meaning and hope too. This example is taken from a one-on-one session; spiritual reminiscence can be done in groups or with individuals:

Interviewer:	When you look back over your life, what things do you remember as times of joy? What times, times of joy? What things were really special things that brought you joy in life?
Jill:	I'm a mother.
Interviewer:	Yes. That says a lot.
Jill:	Well it is a lot.
Interviewer:	Yes, indeed.
Jill:	I would say, and you have got to have a home clean and tidy, and being a mother you've got to have food and lots of things. Be good manager for a start, especially if you have got to go to work to help, look after your families, if you have a family.

(MacKinlay and Trevitt, 2012, p.122)

Many of the older people we worked with in care experienced war in their earlier life. English may be a second language for many of these people, and this may make it hard to communicate as the second language is often lost with increasing dementia. However, the spiritual reminiscence groups can be valuable for helping these people to come to terms with the meaning of their lives. One small group was composed of Latvians, all of whom had come to Australia as displaced persons after World War II. They shared a lot together, of the hard times from their earlier lives, and where they found meaning now:

Sophia said her singing has given her greatest meaning (she was an opera singer), however, lack of money for her training meant that she was only ever in the chorus. Sophia showed the group facilitator a patchwork quilt on her knees that she had made (it was beautiful), and the facilitator attended to it, touching it as Sophia spoke. Sophia told the group that her mother died when she was three. Her older sister looked after her and taught her to read from the newspaper.

Sophia likes poetry, 'I do, I do a lot.' She said that she had it here [the poetry she has written], about 75 pages of it, and suddenly it disappeared. She was visibly upset by this. She said that she cried and cried. She said that she asked her daughter if she took it and she said no. It was all the time in her drawer, but now it is gone. It was in Latvian, so she can't understand why someone else would have taken it. She has read it to a woman in the kitchen, and she said it was beautiful. [It seems she translated it.]

(MacKinlay and Trevitt, 2012, p.144)

Another member of the Latvian group, Paul, reflected on his early life:

> He was a soldier, in the German army. He said: 'My father died when I was seven years old.' Then, he told of being caught in the war. Here, in a new country after the war, he said, nobody liked him – not the Germans, not the Australians. He talked about being in a concentration camp. At another point he remembered the summer festivals in Latvia where they sang and danced all night. He smiled for some time at the memory, and that he had been involved in something adventurous. He did not normally show much emotion.
>
> (MacKinlay and Trevitt, 2012, p.145)

These memories are important, not so much for the cognition involved, but for the meaning to those who remembered now. Where facts are the focus of the session, participants with dementia may become distressed as they feel they are being tested and may fail. However, being engaged with memories of special times of life, such as the examples from the Latvian group above enables the individuals to feel comfortable in sharing. In this group many of their shared memories stirred the memories of the others in their group, as there were numerous connections back to the early and hard times of their lives.

Closure of session

It is important to bring adequate closure to each session. If difficult issues have been raised and/or discussed, deal with these sensitively – the group session for the week is completed by bringing the participants back to a place of hope. If any issues need further support, then with the person's permission a referral can be made to an appropriate person, such as a chaplain, or a counsellor.

Bring the session to closure, re-emphasizing the positive aspects of the life journey.

Thank the group members for sharing and encourage them to return next week.

Chapter 8

Week 2
Relationships, isolation and connecting

Revise and prepare for the session using the guidelines for Part 2.

It is a good idea to begin to prepare for the group before the meeting, with personal reflection on your own life and relationships, then centering and preparing for the way that you might enter into the dialogue.

The emphasis this week is on relationships. Relationship is important for all human beings. Hughes *et al.* (2006, p.35) note 'people with dementia have to be understood in terms of relationships, not because this is all that is left to them, but because this is characteristic of all our lives'. For many older people, with or without dementia, relationship is what provides most meaning in life. Personhood is all about relationships (Kitwood, 1997).

When we asked people with dementia, during their in-depth interviews, where they found meaning, it was most often through relationship. This of course is very much as it is for any human being. The main difference for those with dementia is in those with more advanced dementia, as it becomes more difficult to remember names and exact relationships with significant people in their lives.

In a recent small group session on relationship, one of the participants said that her mother was a wonderful support to her. Suddenly she stopped speaking, and we all waited. A moment later, she said, 'of course, it's not my mother, it's my daughter, but she is like a mother to me' (group session, MacKinlay, 2014). Sometimes they will confuse an adult child for a parent, or talk to an adult child about their own child whom they love, but seem not to realize that they are speaking to that very person. This can be hard for the adult child, who may feel unrecognized, perhaps even discounted, and may wonder what benefit there is in continuing to visit. And yet, it is through relationship that people with dementia are able to connect with others and find meaning in their very existence (MacKinlay and Trevitt, 2012).

Relationships in dementia

Before beginning this week's session, take some time to reflect about the importance of relationship for all human beings.

People with dementia have to be understood in terms of relationships, not because this is all that is left to them, but because this is characteristic of all our lives. (Hughes et al., 2006, p.35)

The research project (MacKinlay and Trevitt 2012) demonstrated that for many people with dementia, relationships were the most important things in their lives, even if past and present were sometimes confused, there was still a sense of 'knowing' and connecting that seemed deep and important to these people. Christine Bryden, diagnosed with early onset dementia said that sometimes she couldn't remember her daughters' names (Bryden, 2012), but she still 'knew' who they were.

Knowing can mean different things. It can be simply having a sense of connectedness with a person, even when names can no longer be associated with the person. The relationship with their parents was in many cases particularly important as was their concern for their partners, either living or dead. Sometimes we can become so focused on whether the person can get the relationships 'right' that we forget that they may be functioning in a different time frame from ours. Some of these matters came out with the question about what gives meaning and the following questions from the second week.

Remember: It is important to mention at each session that what is shared in the group setting stays within the group and is not discussed with other people. It may be helpful to let other staff know the main theme being the focus of each week, in case participants raise issues related to this theme after the group session.

Topics for week 2

What are/have been the best things about relationships in your life?

Use this as a starting point for exploring relationships with the group. You can follow up with *inviting* further dialogue on the topic of relationships, why do you miss (insert name of person or relationship – husband, wife, daughter, son etc)? What special things do you remember about (insert name of person)? Use further dialogue to extend the conversation, as the group members are comfortable.

Think of a number of questions, such as:

- Who visits you?

- Who do you miss?

- Who have you been especially close to?

- Do you have many friends here?

- Who are your friends?

- Do you ever feel lonely? When might you feel lonely? Follow up on things that might be associated with time of day, place etc.

- Do you like to be alone?

We sometimes act as though being with others and interacting with them is important for everyone. But this fails to take into account the differences in personality, and the spiritual resources that some older people have developed. Some older people are also happy in solitude.

Ageing is like a 'natural monastery' (Rick Moody, 1995, p.96).

We don't always need to be 'doing' something. It is sometimes good just to sit and reflect on life.

In the following examples from spiritual reminiscence sessions, you can see the variety of experiences of connecting that the participants have shared. Think about how these examples might guide your own work with spiritual reminiscence.

Facilitator:	So what have been the best things about relationships?
Joe:	Relationships, well for me relationships are, more or less, the anchor the stability peg in my life. In my daily existence I suppose in everything I do. It refers to how does this reflect if I do this how does this reflect on the people around me. My wife, my children, my mother and father not around any more anyway.
Amy:	Well the most important relationship I have is with my mother.
Facilitator:	Do you ever feel lonely Maggie?
Maggie:	No, I miss people. I miss my husband terribly. Um, no I don't feel lonely, if I feel lonely I get up and talk to someone.

(MacKinlay and Trevitt, 2006, p.35–6)

June expresses her feelings about her husband (they were both in residential care) and his rapid cognitive decline:

> So I am just living with him, and doing the best I can. And at one stage, uh, I thought, well, because they ought to make a thing about it, so that he could, or I could have a bit more life with him. But, I just thought, living at the moment, just seeing what the Lord will say to me, and then I will do it.
>
> (MacKinlay and Trevitt, 2006, p.36)

Although relationship is important for human beings, not all people need to be with others all the time; being alone and/or needing company were discussed by some of the participants in the next examples:

> *Daphne:*   I am not a visitor, I am a loner.
>
> *Facilitator:*   You are a loner.
>
> *Daphne:*   They have all invited me, but I, somebody says come and have a cup of coffee with me, my answer is always no thank you.
>
> *Facilitator:*   Oh. Claire, it's hard to catch you I think in the lounge. Do you go to the lounge very often?
>
> *Claire:*   No dear.
>
> *Daphne:*   No, nor do I.
>
> *Facilitator:*   Do you like your room best?
>
> *Claire:*   I am happy there.
>
> (MacKinlay and Trevitt, 2012, p.224)

The research assistant who recorded and kept a journal of the sessions remarked on the group interactions of these people:

> Claire has only one daughter, who visits her. Hetty points to Claire and says, 'she's such a nice person' referring to the daughter. When she realized what she had said could have been ambiguous, she added, pointing again to Claire, 'and so is she.' All participants laugh at this.
>
> They are all attentive to each other and enjoying the conversation. Three group members agree they like their own company and don't mind being alone.
>
> After the group ended, the facilitator said that she was most surprised by Claire. Normally she would not attend social functions or activities, even when encouraged to by staff, but stayed in her room. If she watched TV in the common room she did not engage with others. Now in the group she was sharing and animated in her discussions, and obviously enjoying the conversation and company of the others. The facilitator was amazed at the marked difference.
>
> (MacKinlay and Trevitt, 2012, p.225)

In the following example, the participants were talking about their most important relationships. At times one of them couldn't remember what they were going to say, or had lost the words they wanted to express, the facilitator gently supported them:

> *Hetty:*   I have got the best daughter I could want.
>
> *Facilitator:*   Oh beautiful. That must be a beautiful relationship, very close, daughter and mother.

Hetty:	Oh yes, I don't know, lost my train of thought really.
Facilitator:	Oh lovely. So anybody else want to speak about chatting to people? How you like to chat if you have a visitor or if you go out.
Don:	You have got to have a common interest otherwise you can't really chat about anything.
Louise:	Well I have lots of, they come, the boys come, and you know, it just goes on and on.
Facilitator:	I think you have got a grandchild called Brad, haven't you?
Louise:	Yes. But they are all to me, yes.
Facilitator:	Tell us something about him, tell us about Brad.
Louise:	Brad.
Facilitator:	Your Brad.
Louise:	Oh I don't know whether I could now, really.
Facilitator:	Never mind. Do you know how old he is now?
Louise:	Pardon.
Facilitator:	Do you know how old he is?
Louise:	Oh you have got me now.
Facilitator:	That's okay, I don't know myself.
Louise:	No, no. Oh I can't talk now.
Facilitator:	That's all right, that's lovely. So your sons come to visit you.

(MacKinlay and Trevitt, 2012, pp.225–6)

Notice in the last example, when Louise is invited to talk about her grandson, and then specifically she is asked his age, and she responds: 'No, no. Oh I can't talk now.' It seems she feels uncomfortable, but is reassured by the facilitator. It's an example of people who have dementia being able to talk more about emotional and spiritual topics, but less able to speak of factual topics.

Notice how the facilitator supports Rose in the following conversation. There is sadness in this session. Rose has trouble remembering her sister's address, and maybe some of the details, but the sense of wanting to connect is strong, and illustrates the importance of relationship, or connecting for these people with dementia:

Facilitator:	Beautiful. And Rose?
Rose:	I have only got one sister alive, and my husband and all his family died, and I am the only one living out of that family. I have got a sister, sister in law, she is only, well she is, she has got TB, just got TB, been in hospital and had the operate, says she is going to be all right, but I feel sorry for her because the woman, her husband's gone. She is all alone.
Facilitator:	Where is she living Rose?

Rose:	She lives in Surrey somewhere, I think I have the address but I have forgotten it. Yes, she's a nice girl. She worked for a long time. She married a doctor. She got divorced and she married this doctor, and he died about seven years ago, so she's on her own. But she has got a son of her own, and she has got two, two grandchildren. But she don't make friends very easily, she is a funny girl in some ways.
Facilitator:	Do you feel you would like to support her a little bit?
Rose:	Hmm. She can't come and see me and I can't go and see her [getting upset].
Facilitator:	It's a long way away Rose, isn't it?
Rose:	Yes. I feel she is lonely…

(MacKinlay and Trevitt, 2012, p.227)

Notice the mention of Rose's emotional upset above. Sometimes it is assumed that people must be kept happy in activities and group work, however, sadness and grief and signs of hurt from past events can come out as people reflect on their lives. All of these experiences and emotions are part of life.

These emotions are not to be shut off, but the people expressing their emotions should be supported and heard at these times. We did find in some of the group sessions that one of the participants would reach out to another of the group who was upset, to touch them, to reassure them. These gestures appeared to be well accepted. Remember that all of the people in these groups had dementia; this did not remove their sensitivity to others in distress, in fact they seemed to be very sensitive to the emotions of others in their group. In this way, bonds were able to form between the group members.

Sharing at a deep level about feelings and relationships is an important way of growing connections with others.

Loss of relationship is a common experience for these older people who have dementia. The next example illustrates this:

Amy:	No, I think that is one of the advantages of a place like this, where as if you were at home, like stay at home, if you are, then I think the loneliness could be quite acute, where as here, well if you walk just up and down the corridor for a while, you will meet up with someone you could talk to, or have a joke with, or something.
Facilitator:	So are you saying it is really up to you?
Amy:	Well it is never completely up to one person I suppose, you've got to get that.
Facilitator:	Two way.
Amy:	Yes, but…well I think personal loneliness in your life is something you have to learn to live with, and we all seem to have to face a certain amount of it don't we.

(MacKinlay and Trevitt, 2012, p.232)

Being in a residential aged care facility does not mean that loneliness is not experienced and it can be hard to establish new relationships, as can be seen here:

Facilitator:	What about you Karen, what do you look back on with sadness? When you look back at your life, what do you remember with sadness? What makes you sad?

Karen: That I have nobody. Nobody.

Violet: That can be sad too.

(MacKinlay and Trevitt, 2012, p.233)

The connections between group members, which we have mentioned already can clearly be seen in the following example from a group session, in week 15 of the weekly sessions, by which time, the group members were feeling comfortable with and accepting of each other. Notice how they support each other, and their awareness of each other's needs. Notice also how the facilitator takes quite a back role in the session, allowing the group members to interact; it is their group:

Facilitator: You right? You look very tired, Hetty.

Daphne: Yes.

Facilitator: Would you like me to take you back now?

Hetty: Oh no.

Facilitator: You'll be right?

Claire: Hetty hopes she is going to be okay.

Daphne: Yes, I know there is a lot of them like that.

Claire: She has got that rattly chest.

Daphne: Yes, I know she has.

Facilitator: You are doing well Hetty.

Claire: Each day getting better.

Hetty: Yes.

Daphne: Started to come to the dining table again, which is nice to see, because so many are away.

Facilitator: Oh that's great Hetty, I did not know that.

Daphne: Yes I had not seen her for weeks, a couple of weeks.

Hetty: Sometimes I, I don't feel as good as I could.

Daphne: Some people can get about better than others. I can just manage. A lot of people can't get around very well.

Hetty: I think it is nice how everybody fits here, fits in place.

(MacKinlay and Trevitt, 2012, p.235)

Closure of session

Bring the session to closure, re-emphasizing the positive aspects of the life journey. Thank the group members for sharing and encouraging them to return next week.

Chapter 9

Week 3

Hopes, fears and worries

Revise and prepare for the session using the guidelines for Part 2.

This week's session focuses on discussion about hopes, fears and worries. This can sometimes produce a number of different responses from the participants. Many of the participants talked about worries about the war in Iraq, financial issues or about their families. Some talked about the government or the lack of manners in younger people. One group discussed the situation in Dilli (East Timor) that had been in the news a few years before and identified ways they could provide some assistance. It is worth noting that many people with dementia still engage with the wider world, if it is possible.

Some may even speak of experiences of life from long ago, perhaps of family issues that were distressing, perhaps even experiences of child abuse, remembered, or spoken of for the first time. Sometimes group facilitators may feel uncomfortable when a group member shares something sensitive and personal.

Being heard is an important ingredient in coming to a place of healing and integration of an event and emotions rising from that event. Some of these issues may become quite important for people with dementia. If the person can be heard in the safe setting of a small group, this can be of great value, both to the person whose story it is and to the other members of the small group.

Sometimes a person who has dementia will keep repeating something; it might be that something is troubling them. If they are able to resolve whatever is on their mind, it may be possible to come to closure of that topic, and a sense of peace may emerge. Over time the group members come to trust each other and have entered into a process of caring and sharing with each other. We have found that relationships within the small group are strengthened in these ways.

Often group members will come to learn that some of the disappointments, fears and events that they experienced from earlier life were also experienced by others in their group. This sharing could open the way to affirmation within the group by other group members. One woman spoke of her experience of not being present when her husband died, and two others in the group said they had the same experience, none had spoken about how guilty they had felt before this group session, and each felt affirmed as they realized they were not alone in their experience. Where the person feels heard, the issue may cease to be raised.

Sharing a difficult experience and feeling heard can lead to healing.

Distressing events remembered

Sometimes a person may remember a life event that was distressing, perhaps from a long time ago. Some would say that reminiscence should not venture into allowing such events to be talked about. However, such events may be triggered in the normal course of life activities at any time, perhaps, for example, even when two of three people share over a cup of coffee. Giving the opportunity for sharing distressful life events in a safe environment can be a healing experience for the person who has shared. It can also be a time of special sharing and bonding within the group. It is not a counselling event, but simply a time of listening and sharing together.

As facilitator, when distressing events are raised:
- *listen attentively*
- *do not judge*
- *be present to the person who is sharing, using appropriate body language*
- *give them adequate time to express their story*
- *affirm the confidentiality of the group setting*
- *do not feel you need to provide a solution or answer, or even do something, simply being heard is all that is necessary in the small group setting*
- *offer referral to counselling if desired.*

It is important that as facilitator you do not attempt to counsel the person, but allow them to speak, listen with attention and be present to them, indicating this by facial expression and body language. Simply feeling heard may mean that the thing spoken of may lose its power to haunt the person (Coleman, 1999) and it can be incorporated into the whole life story of the person. Such an experience may lead to healing of some past distresses or anxieties. Should there be something that the speaker finds hard to deal with, it is important to follow up with referral to counsellors as needed, outside of the group time.

In an earlier study of cognitively intact older people about 70 per cent of the participants named dementia as a potential fear for the future. In contrast, the participants in our study had dementia, and it was generally not named as a fear (MacKinlay, 2001). Generally the people with dementia in our studies seemed less worried than their cognitively competent contemporaries.

Topics for week 3

What are your hopes and fears for the future?

- What things do you worry about?

- Do you have any fears? What about?

- Do you feel you can talk to anyone about things that trouble you?

- What gives you hope now?

    - Perhaps your faith brings hope.

    - Perhaps your hope is through your family.

    - Perhaps your hope…(read through book to check out possible sources of hope).

The following responses were to the facilitator question:

Do you have any fears? Or worries?

A variety of responses were given to these invitations to share:

Ivy:	Well, actually I haven't any fear – real fear – except to make sure my family is well – and now we've got hope – I hope that Ron and I are together until one of us departs this life but I hope my family down the coast – are well and happy and that's about all it think.
Ruby:	Yes, I fear – there's a lot to fear in the world today – that does worry me – there's nothing I can do about it – but fear – I'm not fearful of anything now.
Bob:	Well, worry, you do worry about the local things a lot – I mean the parliaments – they made an awful mess – I feel that we could do better if we were there – but I doubt it – because it's very confusing now the way everyone's in it – and you vote for somebody and he turns out to be no good.
Facilitator:	What gives you hope now?
Ivy:	Yes well I hope these boys grow up; both their boys grow up as good as their fathers are, that's my greatest hope. The best thing of all is that I get on so well with their wives.
Facilitator:	So what is it that gives you hope in life now?
James:	I hope to be able to continue on in life for a little while, helping anyone that I can.
Jenny:	I'm hopeless.

Facilitator:	What do you mean?
May:	We are all full of hope for you.

(MacKinlay and Trevitt, 2006, p.37)

Health featured as perhaps the most important topic of worry for these people. But, importantly in the following excerpt, notice that the interviewer speaks little and encourages Don to continue to express his thoughts, concerns and feelings:

Don:	The most important thing I worry about is lack of, uh, my own intention to do anything.
Interviewer:	Mmm hmm
Don:	Because when you are in a place like this, you just have to carry out the rules and regulations, and allow things to take their course.
Interviewer:	Mmm
Don:	Whereas when if I was on my own as I was for some time before I came in here, I could go and come as I liked. I could eat or not eat as I liked.
Interviewer:	Mmm
Don:	And in that way my initiative was not undermined.
Interviewer:	Mmm, mmm
Don:	But there is no such thing as initiative here. It is all rules and regulations. And if you try to be insistent, you upset the whole system, and that doesn't do anybody any good. And uh, and I have had one or two bad spells of health, which has uh, knocked me down quite a lot. In fact I am just recovering from a bit of pneumonia.
Interviewer:	Mmm
Don:	But thank goodness it is passing away.
Interviewer:	It is settled?
Don:	So, that is one of the things which was telling on me really much when I first came in here.
Interviewer:	Mmm
Don:	But by the help of people of the church, particularly who came around to see me, and knew me from the days that I was able to… Also the biggest problem I have is that my sight failed.

(MacKinlay and Trevitt, 2012, p.128)

> What kinds of strategies can you use to encourage the person to share what is on their heart and mind?

A sense of hope and acceptance was seen among a number of the participants, as in this example:

When asked by the facilitator, 'What gives you hope now?'

Hetty: Well, I am ready to go.
              I have lived all my life.
              And I am not worried about going.

(MacKinlay and Trevitt, 2012, p.158)

In another conversation the following was heard, as Daphne was given space to reflect on her life journey:

Facilitator: Wonderful, that's wonderful. Okay. A number of these things we have actually talked about it various things already, right, well what is it that gives you hope in life now?

Daphne: Oh, only that.

Facilitator: Only that?

Daphne: Yes. Well, I mean I have achieved, I feel I have achieved all I can achieve in this world, that is how I feel. I have worked hard at many professions and, or just ordinary blue-collar work if you like, put it that way.
              I have worked in factories, I have been successful in that, and had control of a room full of people working making shoes, and over here I was in the public service, I came back all right after all that ordeal, got back and did more and more examinations, as you do, to go up the ladder as it were, and that is how I did, and I got promotions to, a promotion to Sydney, after eight years being in Hobart, and I was only there six years, and somebody from Canberra learned I was studying, what is the name of the course, ah, not bookkeeping, more than that, the whole…

(MacKinlay and Trevitt, 2012, p.158)

In a number of sessions participants reflected on their hope and faith, as in the following example:

Eve: I suppose I want to be the person, that I, would choose to be.

Facilitator: Yes.

Evelyn: Uh, I mean we can't all do the things the right way I know, but I would like to be, uh, I don't think I would want to be a great biblical you know, reader or whatever, but I would like to, do my bit for God, you know, and, or for anyone, if there was a need for, you know, support for someone or something like that.

Graham: My hope for the Lord is, do the best I can with what I have got.

Facilitator: What gives you hope, now?

Candy: Christianity I think, that is a hope. My hope, other people have different ideas.

Facilitator: So what is it that gives you hope in life now?

Nancy: I am just hoping to meet as many people as I can, uh to, to get this message through, because I know that God means me to do it.

I know what he wants.

And death, I just wait, because he said those who wait upon the Lord will rise up like an eagle.

(MacKinlay and Trevitt, 2012, pp.160–1)

On the other hand, not all of the participants found hope; some had no sense of hope. This was not necessarily related to their dementia, but could have been associated with personality and other factors related to growing older.

For example Margaret, in a one-on-one session of spiritual reminiscence:

Margaret has kept her desire not to be admitted to a residential facility a secret from her children, believing it was 'for the best'. Her increasing frailty and a fall and fracture all gave added weight to the case for residential care.

Margaret: Well there's no hope.

Interviewer: There's no hope?

Margaret: I've just got to go on. Hmm, that's what I think anyhow. The family have put me here, I didn't want to come, but I didn't tell them that. This is the best I think. Because I fall over. I fell and broke my wrist and that started it all off.

Interviewer: Yes and you really feel that you can't manage by yourself anymore.

Margaret: No.

Interviewer: Yeah it's a hard decision isn't it?

Margaret: Hmm. Yes it is, it is a hard decision, but once you've made it you've got to go through with it I think.

(MacKinlay and Trevitt, 2012, p.165)

> In the example above, think how you might respond to Margaret and her inability to find hope in her present situation.

The problem of memory and hope is shown here. Jessica was asked about where she found hope and for her it was about working hard to remember things:

Jessica: Remembering things.

Interviewer: That gives you hope, remembering things?

Jessica: Yes.

Interviewer: So you try and remember things?

Jessica: Keep playing them to retain them.

(MacKinlay and Trevitt, 2012, p.164)

Talking about hopes, fears and worries is also likely to raise questions about dying and death. This week's theme was likely to raise some of these discussions. Death and dying were subjects openly spoken of in the groups, with a number of participants simply accepting death as part of life. In several groups a group member died between one week's session and the next. Dealing with this was just part of the normal routine, in the following example, Mary was easily able, with the facilitator's support to begin to work with her grief following the death of her companion:

Facilitator: Are there any, we have had a bit of a hard week I think here haven't we Mary?

Mary: In what way?

Facilitator: Well we have lost Stan this week. Did you remember? That he died on Sunday. And we don't have Joyce because today – the funeral is on, and she has gone with her daughter. So there is some hard thing about living here isn't there?

Mary: Well I think it is a sad place to live, to stay, I do.

Facilitator: Is that because you are near the end of your life, and is that the reason do you think.

[Voices talking over each other.]

Mary: There are all old people here and there is something wrong with most of them.

Mary: No I get down sometimes I am the biggest downer.

Facilitator: I wonder if I can get – would it help in that circumstance if when lost somebody, it doesn't matter how that would be – would it make it any easier if you knew that they were ready to die? How would you feel if you knew that personally? Wouldn't it make it easier?

Mary: Oh no, you would miss them terribly. No I don't think it would make it any easier. It might at the time you might think their time is up, but not really. You've got the rest of your life to live you don't know when you're going to slip off. We've got to go I know that, I can't think of anything.

Facilitator: That's a big statement that's nice, did you want to say anything about that Mary?

Mary: No, not really.

Facilitator: Does it help when you lose somebody if you knew they were ready?

Mary: Oh yes it would, certainly would.

Facilitator: Would it make it any easier for whom, for you?

Mary: Might be it would I think the best thing of all would be to go suddenly.

Facilitator: Well I think that in Stan's case he did go suddenly didn't he? He was with us, suddenly he was gone.

(MacKinlay and Trevitt, 2012, pp.175–6)

Closure of session

Be sensitive to any issues that have been raised in the group setting, remembering that it is not necessary to 'fix' things, but rather, the aim is to hear the person and to respond to them in affirmation. It may be necessary to take up some matters with chaplaincy, or counselling with the participant's agreement. Bring the session to closure, re-emphasizing the positive aspects of the life journey. Thank the group members for sharing and encourage them to return next week.

Self-care for the facilitator is important and debriefing and professional or peer supervision need to be available.

Chapter 10

Week 4

Growing older and transcendence

Revise and prepare for the session using the guidelines for Part 2.

One of the benefits of spiritual reminiscence is that it allows people to think about the changes they have experienced in growing older, whether physical changes, like having less energy, disabilities or psychosocial changes such as role changes and/or losses. It is also helpful to reflect on how they are managing these changes and any difficulties they may be having, as well as the degree of transcendence they have achieved.

What is important in life is not what losses we have experienced or disabilities and chronic diseases we live with, but how we manage to live with these. It may be that through experiences of adversity or suffering, the person has grown in their spiritual life. Their sharing of these episodes of life may be strengthening for others in the group as well. In a very real sense, the development of transcendence is more than a coping mechanism; it is a letting go and an experiencing of new depths of what it means to be human.

Resources

Resources for this session may include examples of the changing body, perhaps photos of activities they used to engage in, perhaps sports, or particular interests of these people. Two examples that came from group members over time were mountain climbing and opera singing. Gardening is an activity that many older people have engaged in; some may still be gardening. It may be helpful to set up preparation for this the week beforehand: resources may trigger conversation about body changes in later life. Even without such prompts, this topic has always elicited much conversation in the sessions.

Topics for week 4

- What's it like growing older?

- Do you have any health problems?

- Do you have memory problems? If so how does that affect what you want to do?

- What are the hardest things in your life now?

- Do you like living here? What's it like living here? Was it hard to settle in? (You can add other questions of a similar kind as appropriate.)

- As you reach the end of your life what do you hope for now?

- What do you look forward to?

Questions about what it is like growing older are a good starting point for this week's session:

Interviewer:	What is it like growing older?
Anita:	I think it takes a while to get to used to it. It's freedom [laughs].

(MacKinlay and Trevitt, 2012, p.94)

In the dialogues below, there didn't seem to be any differences between what the participants talked about and what a small group of people who did not have dementia might talk about. However, if the conversation had stayed at a purely factual level, without engaging with emotions and the spiritual, these people might have been less able to take part.

Facilitator:	What was the hardest thing in your life, now what's the hardest thing?
Ivy:	Now, I don't think I have a hardest thing. I suppose it's been not having the family around me. I love having the boys at home and the girls. No, I don't think I have got any problems.
Ruby:	Not seeing.
Facilitator:	Yeah.
Ruby:	I am very blind and it's got worse it keeps getting worse too. And being deaf as well doesn't help.
Facilitator:	Bob what's it like growing older? You had good health?
Bob:	I have had reasonably good health, but you reach a point when you are growing older that you start to lose the sharpness. That's what I found, and you are inclined to worry about the stuff that you can't remember. The thing that makes you think is your health, and the security and what you are going to do when you reach an age when you can't look after yourself.
Facilitator:	What was it like growing older? How do you feel about that?
Jane:	I found it quite pleasant, new experiences, new people, new places. I have not minded it.
Facilitator:	So Mary what do you think it is like growing older?
Mary:	I don't like it. Definitely not, everything seems to stop.

You can't do the things you used to do, don't take any notice of me.

Facilitator:	My next question is do you like living here?
Ivy:	I don't have to cook, I don't have to wash.
Facilitator:	Do you have any memory problems?
Ivy:	A little bit, like I won't remember yesterday, further back yes, but I forget the bit that just happened. Otherwise I am all right.

The following exchange arose without a question from the facilitator and occurred in a group that had been running for four months:

June:	[Speaking of her husband.] He's just losing his memory. It's one of those things.
May:	Well he doesn't want mine. It's an awful thing though when you don't remember yourself.
Facilitator:	Yes it is a shame isn't it, and it's hard for June.

(MacKinlay and Trevitt, 2006, pp.38–9)

This is another good example of the conversation on this topic, with plenty of engagement of the participants:

Facilitator:	Okay, what's it like growing older?
Rose:	Ooh, what's it like growing older?
Facilitator:	Yes.
Rose:	Ohh.
Hetty:	Well you have got to make the best of it.
Daphne:	Mmm.
Hetty:	Forget about getting older.
Daphne:	Forget about it.
Rose:	You can't do things you want to do when you get older, like go dancing.
Claire:	I'm loving it.
Facilitator:	Loving it, well, party girl talking.
Hetty:	I never thought I'd get to ninety.
Facilitator:	That's not very old is it?
Daphne:	You are ninety.
Hetty:	Yes.
Daphne:	Yes.
Hetty:	And I never thought I would get there.

Daphne:	Mmm.
Hetty:	My family, the young ones, reckon I will get to one hundred.
Facilitator:	Get to one hundred?
Hetty:	Yes.
Facilitator:	Yes, I reckon you will.
Rose:	I don't want to live to one hundred.
Hetty:	No, I don't particularly.
Rose:	You have to go the way you want to get out.
Hetty:	One hundred…
Rose:	One hundred, oh right.
Facilitator:	It's a high number, isn't it.
Daphne:	I think it is true for most of us, that as we get older we get weaker, in one way or another. Some people cannot hear, some can't see, some can't walk, all those sorts of things beset us, which we have not experienced before, because we can always do plenty just when and where we like. Can't do it anymore, dependent upon somebody else very often.
Facilitator:	Mmm. Somebody else's eyes, or somebody else's ears, or somebody else's hands. Is that right?

(MacKinlay and Trevitt, 2012, pp.94–5)

From these examples, it is easy to see that the participants are at different stages of self-transcendence in the process of growing older. Some show wisdom and self-forgetting while others continue to focus on their physical health.

Daphne was one participant who did appear to have reflected on what lay ahead and showed some self-transcendence:

Daphne:	Just thinking about the future, and the future for me, is to go and, uh, at one time, when he is ready, uh, put me into, um, a place that he has prepared for me.
Facilitator:	Yes.
Daphne:	And this is really my whole heart, the other is just struggling along, as you will find most of us are… So I manage very well, but um, when you say what is the greatest thing, in a way there is not anything on earth because I just think that my journey is almost to the end, and I am hoping it is, uh, not, not, I was depressed last week, not very often I am, but what with the kitchen and everything else being out of order, and everyone being at their wits end, and not knowing what's where, and it's um, I do feel, a lot better this week, and I have got back to normal again now.

(MacKinlay and Trevitt, 2012, p.97)

In an individual session of spiritual reminiscence faith was acknowledged to provide strength in keeping going as well as still having a responsibility to another person (his wife):

Graham: Pardon me. The good things. Peace with God.

Interviewer: Yes.

Graham: Relationship with the Lord, holding onto that firm. That's another point of mine. Well if I can't expose everything or see it, and quite often I can't, I have got to, what pardon me, I have got to acknowledge a lot of other things, and I have to care for Audrey my wife, to see how she is going.

(MacKinlay and Trevitt, 2012, p.107)

Closure of session

Bring the session to closure, re-emphasizing the positive aspects of the life journey. Thank the group members for sharing and encourage them to return next week.

Chapter 11

Week 5
Spiritual and religious beliefs

Revise and prepare for the session using the guidelines for Part 2.

This week is an exploration of spiritual and religious beliefs. Do be aware that some participants may not normally use the term 'spirituality' and it may be better to stay with the language of meaning, rather than use the word 'spiritual'. It may be of value to include some religious or spiritual symbols or objects, being aware of the background of the group members. Music or art, or craft signifying spiritual aspects can be helpful too.

Response to meaning may be in many forms, through worship, through art, music, poetry, through symbols, drama, prayer, and reading of sacred texts. Symbols may be religious or secular. There is something about human beings that brings a deep seated need for connections through symbol and ritual. For those who have no connections with anything of a religious nature, symbols still retain their importance.

The importance of symbols lies in their ability to carry meaning for the particular people of a particular culture. Thus the variety of symbols is only restricted by the imagination of the people involved. Effective symbols can be flowers, leaves, pebbles, water, candles, religious symbols, a cross for Christians, prayer mats for Muslims, incense, rosaries, statues for Hindus and Buddhists. Special foods, fasting and ceremonies would fit here too, such as the Muslim observance of Ramadan, and special Jewish festivals (Abdalla and Patel, 2010; Barzaghi, 2010; Cohen, 2010; Rayner and Bilimoria, 2010 in MacKinlay and Trevitt, 2012).

Each group or cohort of older people has experienced different social and religious practices in their families or origin. At this time we are seeing the older baby boomers retiring and some will be starting to need aged care services. There are real differences between the baby boomer cohort of people and those who were in the cohort before them. Those in their seventies or older were brought up in an era when there was a greater participation in religious life.

The baby boomers being born after WWII (1946–1965) have vastly different experiences of growing up. Well known are the social and educational differences for this cohort of the population, perhaps a little less well known is that this was the first group in many western countries where there was not an expectation of church and Sunday school attendance. So, unlike the previous cohort of older people, numbers of the ageing baby boomer generation will have limited or perhaps no experience of religious faith.

The baby boomers have also been more likely than previous generations to explore religions other than Christianity. Further, migrations of people of different faith and cultural backgrounds in this age group will add even greater variety to the beliefs and practices of these people. Therefore a lower proportion of baby boomers, who require residential care, will probably want denominational religious services. However, a recent study of baby boomer future needs in spirituality and spiritual care (MacKinlay and Burns, 2013, unpublished) has shown that spirituality is important to this group of older people. Thus spiritual reminiscence, as a valuable means of finding meaning in life, will continue to have an important role for these people, as they grow older.

Some may wish to explore religious faith as they grow older, others may not; the opportunity to explore religious faith as well as the broader perspectives of spirituality should be available. It is interesting to talk about the meaning of God or a deity with these groups. The facilitator needs to feel comfortable with raising and talking about these topics.

During this week themes explore participants' early memories of church. Some participants described walking miles to church, or going to church when they were five years old with their parents. For those who do not have a religious background, questions about where they receive spiritual support or if they seek this support can be asked.

Some older people may not relate to the term 'spiritual'; be prepared for this by using other words that may express what 'spiritual' means. For instance, you might ask about beliefs and values that they hold, and what the deepest things in their lives are.

We have found it valuable to ask what they think God is like. This does not seem to be a question that causes distress to participants; it is a way into the topic, and people may feel free to say at this point, they do not believe there is a God, or they may let you know what their negative thought about God are. Or they may express their sense and understanding of a God of Love. Knowing what the person thinks and feels in response to this question is an important starting point for pastoral and spiritual care. This care is not only religious care but is far broader.

Topics for week 5

- What do you think God is like?

- Do you have an image of God or some sense of a deity or otherness?

- If you hold an image of God, can you tell me about this image?

- Do you feel near to God?

- What are your earliest memories of church, mosque, temple or other worship?

- As a child, did you go to Sunday school, church or take part in any other religious or spiritual activities?

- Where do you go to get spiritual support?

- Who is the most important person to give you spiritual support?

- Do you find art or music expresses spirituality for you?

- Do you find plants, gardens, or animals are ways of expressing spirituality for you?

The ways that we respond to our deepest spiritual needs and desires do not diminish as we grow older, some say they may even be intensified. It is important that older people with dementia, like any other older people, are able to engage with meaningful activities, or even quietly contemplate life as they desire. Beliefs and values as well as culture and personal choice influence the ways that people will want to engage with spiritual needs. Religious worship will be among this variety. The liturgy and the Holy Communion or the Eucharist may be a vitally important connecting point for Christians, even when speech has been lost.

In this week's theme, these areas are explored through a range of topics. It is important that as a facilitator you are able to feel comfortable in sharing with participants of different faiths and none, and that you are able to respectfully listen and support group members in their explorations of spiritual and religious beliefs.

Examples will help you to find ways to easily open up conversations on these deeper topics, and to feel confident in introducing topics you might not have used in the past. Notice also how the participants respond to the invitation to share.

Facilitator:	George, how do you see God? What is God to you?
George:	He is to me what he is in my heart, and in my mind.
Facilitator:	You do you think of God as?
Frank:	Yeah he is above us.
Annie:	Someone omnipotent.
Facilitator:	Yeah, what was that? I missed what you said sorry.
Annie:	God is omnipotent in my book.
Frank:	I think God is there to care for us.
Facilitator:	I think that is really good.
Jess:	Yeah he is there and whatever the time comes he is there. Whenever we need help we know, we pray.
Facilitator:	Have you got a special relationship with him?
Annie:	It always seems to be where he guides me. In what direction, and I feel that God has turned me that way for what reason.
Facilitator:	What are your earliest memories of church?
John:	My father was an organist and I used to pump the organ for him… I was too young to understand where I was, I would be about three or four.

(MacKinlay and Trevitt, 2006, p.41)

One example of relationship with God was expressed by this woman when asked by the facilitator: 'So do you feel near to God now, Elma?' Elma replied: 'God and I have developed, he is always here' (MacKinlay and Trevitt, 2012, p.239).

Staff sometimes hesitate to ask or to even introduce topics related to religious faith, or even spirituality – even understood in its broadest terms, as it is in this program.

It is important to introduce topics in such a way that group participants will not feel uncomfortable and will want to engage in the conversation.

The following examples give information about the way these people see their religious faith and are therefore very helpful in working with each person in supporting their spiritual view points and needs. In the excerpt below, the interviewer moved from another topic to introduce the topic of faith. Note how this was done:

Interviewer: I'd like to take a change in direction now and ask you, do you have a faith then?

Jane: I'm Church of England.

Interviewer: Yes.

Jane: I go to Bible studies.

Interviewer: Yes.

Jane: I don't go every week. I don't practise faith every week but when I… I go.

Interviewer: Now you say you enjoy going to church and so you go to the services here?

Jane: Yes, they have the services on Sunday. They're there. The services are very nice.

(MacKinlay and Trevitt, 2012, p.241)

A change of religious faith is seen in the following excerpts, the first is from an initial interview, while the second is from a later group session:

Interviewer: Now I want to take a change of where we are going at the moment, and I want to ask you about whether you have any sense or image of God or some kind of deity or otherness?

Rose: No I haven't. I used to. [Mumbles.]

Interviewer: And what happened?

Rose: I couldn't, I didn't take [pause] I can't speak as well as I used to speak.

Interviewer: Do you go to any of the services here?

Rose:	Yes I go every Friday morning.
Interviewer:	And do you enjoy those?
Rose:	Yes.
Interviewer:	Well that's good.
Rose:	I don't feel the same about it.
Interviewer:	You don't feel the same about it? Okay, can you tell me a little bit more about how you feel about that now?
Rose:	Oooh, to tell you the truth I haven't even thought about that.
Interviewer:	You have not really thought about that very much.
Rose:	No, not since I have been here, I used to do, I used to go to church, and I was very good. When I was little I used to go to church every Sunday.
Interviewer:	That was just part of what you did on Sunday.
Rose:	Yes.
Interviewer:	So is there a way in which you miss that now?
Rose:	Mmm hmm, it's not the same anymore.
Interviewer:	No, so do you see that you have any spiritual needs?
Rose:	Not at the moment.
Interviewer:	Not at the moment. Now I am wondering if you have, you say you go to the church services here on a Friday?
Rose:	Some weeks, also on the weekend.
Interviewer:	Yes, on a Friday.
Interviewer:	Do you have any negative memories about anything to do with religion at all?
Rose:	Yes I used to go out at Sunday, I used to like to go to church, on Christmas and Boxing Day.
Rose:	I used to be good, I used to go to church and I used to do things with friends, and go to church, I used to enjoy it.
Interviewer:	Would you like to be able to do that again? Be able to enjoy church?
Rose:	I think it will come back to me.
Interviewer:	You think?
Rose:	It could come back to me.
Interviewer:	Would you like the chaplain to come and visit you.
Rose:	I don't know him do I?

Interviewer:	Hmmm?
Rose:	I don't know him very well.
Interviewer:	Well there is a lady chaplain here at the moment.
Rose:	Here? In the church here?

(MacKinlay and Trevitt, 2012, pp.243–4)

Rose has continued her concern expressed in the initial interview, in one of the group sessions:

Facilitator:	Anyone else want to say whether this group's made a difference from the way you feel about God?
Rose:	I don't know, but I think I seldom to go but I don't know when. I've gone from one to the other. I used to go to church and all, but I don't know what's stopping me, I got ill or something and…
Facilitator:	Can you express Rose, thank you for being so honest, um can you, would you like to say ah you've gone from one to the other, where do you want to be, do you know?
Rose:	Well I want to go back to where I was.
Facilitator:	Which is where?
Rose:	Oh I used to be happy, I used to, I used to pray and everything else, but I don't pray now.
Facilitator:	Do you mean, are you saying that you would like to start praying again?
Rose:	Yes, but I, something has stopped me, I don't know what it is, but it does.

(MacKinlay and Trevitt, 2012, p.252)

Following the end of this session the following is recorded from the research assistant's journal:

When tape turned off, the facilitator offers to pray for Rose. She says 'yes' and appears to be grateful and moved by this, crying more openly.

The group holds hands and the facilitator leads the group in prayer.

They stay for a while talking about the freedom they feel in being able to talk with each other and how they feel close to each other in faith.

(MacKinlay and Trevitt, 2012, p.253)

Closure of session

Be aware that a number of very different experiences may have been shared in this session. Affirm the group members in their individual ways of expressing their spiritual beliefs. Bring the session to closure, re-emphasizing the positive aspects of the life journey. Thank the group members for sharing and encourage them to return next week.

Chapter 12

Week 6
Spiritual and religious practices

This session focuses on the final of the six weekly themes of the model of Spiritual Tasks and Process of Ageing. After this session the themes begin at the first weekly theme again.

Revise and prepare for the session using the guidelines for Part 2.

Preparation for the session

Prepare before the session for the time of meeting, reflecting in the way that suits you as a facilitator. It may be of value to include some religious or spiritual symbols or objects, being aware of the background of the group members. Thus sacred texts may be part of the resources provided, according to the faith of the participants. Religious symbols, again, choose these according to the faiths of the group members. Some groups may have humanist members, and symbols, such as candles or flowers may be appropriate. Music or art, or craft signifying spiritual aspects can be helpful too.

The discussion this week revolves around the activities that the participants are presently involved in. In our study, all the participants were in residential aged care, however, many older people will be in community groups, and their interests and activities will vary greatly.

It is important to focus on what is relevant to the needs of these particular people. Some residents attended activities, studies, prayer groups, or services of worship weekly, others declared that they were Christians but did not attend organized activities or services. In a study of ageing baby boomers, meditation was listed as one of their spiritual activities (MacKinlay and Burns, unpublished study 2013). Data from previous cohorts of older people showed that few of them had any experience of meditation. This is likely to be different as the baby boomers grow older.

The theme of this session is a good opportunity to identify what people's spiritual and/or religious needs are and whether these needs are being met. Many report prayer and reading the Bible as a part of their spiritual practices. For those participants who express their spirituality through music, art, pets, the environment, or any kind of creativity, ask what they do now and what they would like to do, to meet these needs.

Topics for week 6

- Do you take part in any religious/spiritual activities now? For example, do you:

    - attend church services

    - take part in Bible studies

    - take part in other religious readings

    - pray

    - meditate or

    - attend study groups?

- Are there particular cultural and/or religious beliefs that should be considered in your care?

- How important are these to you?

- How can we help you to find meaning now?

As with the week 5 theme, this week may also be one where the facilitator may be unsure how to open up the conversation. It is important that he or she is comfortable in speaking about religion and spirituality. The following example is taken from individual one-on-one interviews, where the interviewer has met the person for the first time:

Interviewer: Mmm, I'm wondering, now do you, do you read any religious things or do you take part in any Bible studies or, um meditation or…

Amy: Yes, well of course prayer is a form of meditation really isn't it.

Interviewer: Yes.

Amy: And er [pause] I try to stay as close to God as I possibly can.

Interviewer: Yes, that is good.

(MacKinlay and Trevitt, 2012, p.241)

Discussion about activities in one group session led to the proposition that grace be held before meals.

Annie: I think it is terrible that we all sit down to these wonderful [meals], and there are people in the world starving, children. And we sit down and hoe in without a word of thanks.

(MacKinlay and Trevitt, 2006, p.43)

The following question elicited a meaningful response – it is only the individual who can find meaning, and relationship is central to this. However, facilitators and other carers may support and assist older people in finding meaning:

Facilitator: How can we help you to find meaning now? Is there any way at all?

Peter: No I have found my meaning.

Facilitator:	Yes, you have your meaning.
Peter:	Yes, you know I am going about it as long as I do, and I want to be friends.

(MacKinlay and Trevitt, 2006, p.43)

Church attendance has often been seen as the only aspect of spirituality or religion, but as can be seen here, it is an important part for some, but certainly not all.

Facilitator:	Yes, so do you take part in the church services here?
Amy:	Oh yes, I go to all of them.
Facilitator:	And do you find them, do you enjoy going?
Amy:	Well, um, it's a hard question to answer because to enjoy is not what the faith is for.
Facilitator:	Okay.
Amy:	It's ah, well probably it is [laugh].
Facilitator:	[laugh] Well yeah okay it, it's more complex than that.
Amy:	[pause] Put it that way.

(MacKinlay and Trevitt, 2012, p.254)

Margaret does not go to church, but takes part in Bible studies:

Margaret:	Oh yes, we all went to Sunday school when we were little.
Interviewer:	Yes.
Margaret:	And then church. Then I got away from church, but I like the Bible studies.
Interviewer:	Yes.
Margaret:	I'm not against, well I am against religion, I don't like religion just like it is.

(MacKinlay and Trevitt, 2012, p.255)

Louise did not attend church or pray, yet took part in the spiritual reminiscence group sessions and appeared comfortable in her participation. The following is from her initial interview:

Interviewer:	Now do you have really early memories in your life of say going to church or Sunday school or something like that?
Louise:	Yes, I used to do that.
Interviewer:	And was that good?
Louise:	Yes it was. I don't do it now.
Interviewer:	No? Do you go to any church services here?
Louise:	Well I could I am sure, and might if I think, I have got a terrible pain of it, if I, kneel in fact, yes.
Interviewer:	Yes. So you have got a pain in your knee?

Louise:	Yes, yes it is now. Talking it does.
Interviewer:	So, do you take part, do you pray, or?
Louise:	Beg your pardon?
Interviewer:	Do you pray, or do you read any religious things at all?
Louise:	No, I don't.

(MacKinlay and Trevitt, 2012, p.255)

Jill, in an in-depth interview, was clear in her opinions about church, and her beliefs were respected.

Interviewer:	Right. And you don't go to church or anything now?
Jill:	No, that's right. I found a lot of wrongs I didn't agree with. Everybody does that though.

(MacKinlay and Trevitt, 2012, p.245)

John had a more nuanced view of religion, supporting his wife, in attending church, but 'not taking it seriously' himself. He was another participant who did not find religious activities or beliefs to be important. At the same time, he appeared happy to be in a group of participants, some of whom had a religious faith, while others in the same group did not. Religious beliefs were discussed openly and respect was given to the different perspectives of the participants.

John:	Well I've read in a religious area like err atmosphere, and it wasn't until I was 16 or 17 that I shed it all and I forced my way through work and everything else, and then I had six years away. And I saw things during those six years that made me wonder, because one minute you're with your mates and the next minute you're burying them and all that sort of thing. And I've been quite cynical about it ever since, I worry about the family of course, but err religion with me, I go with Joyce to church and appreciate it, but I don't take it seriously. Um, but err I'm not being funny about this but…
Facilitator:	Thank you it's very kind of you to share.
John:	I find it hard to um, because there's things I've seen that I could never reconcile with religion, there's too much and I can see it now. It's one of those lasting impressions of what you've seen and that and err.
	And err I follow a life which is guided by principles and I appreciate people who are religious and all that sort of thing, but it doesn't affect me.
	I love my girl and she can be very religious at times, but we go to church together, but err no I can't. I couldn't get up and spruik [speak publicly, evangelize or promote] about it or anything like that, because I would say that I am being a damn hypocrite.

(MacKinlay and Trevitt, 2012, p.245)

In one of the individual interviews, Brenda spoke of her reasons for attending church:

Interviewer:	And I wonder if I could ask you, do you have a faith or a belief in your life? Do you have a belief system?
Brenda:	No. I am very. What can you say, what can you call me.
	I am very anti all the religious stuff. And I really believe that people overdo it, and if they just get on with their own things, we'd all be far better off.
Interviewer:	Right.
Brenda:	That's why [pause] oh I mean I still go to church.
Interviewer:	Oh do you?
Brenda:	I still go to church because, in Durham, a church school. So I still go, but only for the singing.
Interviewer:	And you really enjoy that?
Brenda:	Yes, and I really enjoy that, yes.

For this group of older people, meditation was not generally part of religious practice, although this is changing with the ageing of baby boomers, whose spiritual and religious practice are often different from the preceding cohort of older people, as discussed earlier.

Facilitator:	Now um, so you go to church services here.
	Do you take part in any Bible studies, or Bible readings or?
Bronwyn:	Yes.
Facilitator:	Yes?
Bronwyn:	Quite a few days I do Bible reading.
Facilitator:	And do you do any meditation at all?
Bronwyn:	I think a lot.
Facilitator:	You think a lot. Yes, within yourself.
Bronwyn:	Yes.

(MacKinlay and Trevitt, 2012, p.247)

Spiritual and religious practices differed, and are likely to be different for different participants in any small groups, but knowing what practices work for people is of value in providing relevant spiritual and pastoral care:

Facilitator:	Anybody attend any prayer groups, or do prayer as a group?
Claire:	Not now, I miss it very much. I used to go every Monday evening used to be the prayer meeting, and those sort of things, yes I do miss but, I carry them in my memory and in my mind and in my spiritual being and it still means a lot to me cause I can remember so much of the past.
Facilitator:	Do you take part in any spiritual or religious activity?

Margaret: Well I don't, but I like Bible study, that's about all that I like now. And um I don't think I'm learning a lot about it, but it's interesting.

     I don't go to church err I don't know why, I did up till the late years, then I dropped out when things went wrong and um I've never been back to church really to enjoy it. But Bible study I like.

Facilitator: Would you like to say how often you do that?

Margaret: Well only here once a week I think it is.

(MacKinlay and Trevitt, 2012, p.244)

Prayer was an important topic in this theme:

Facilitator: So, about prayer, do you all pray?

Amy: Yes.

Facilitator: Yep.

Amy: Everyday.

Facilitator: Yes.

Ben: Yes.

Facilitator: Do you pray Ben?

Ben: Not so much that I used to.

Facilitator: Yes, what about you Anita?

Anita: I keep him pretty busy.

Facilitator: Hmmm, yes.

     What about you Anita, do you um, do you say a set pray when you pray, or do you just bring whatever is on your mind?

Anita: I just sort of talk.

Amy: Talk to God I call it, talking to God it should be really. When things get really bad I wonder whether he is listening, you know, where are you God?

Facilitator: Yes, that's when you cry out, isn't it?

Anita: I wish there was more opportunities for myself, and in fact I could ask for myself, you know, I visit in my mind. Do you see? Yes I do that.

(MacKinlay and Trevitt, 2012, p.250)

Facilitator: Claire, would, how would you feel if someone came to pray with you? Would you like that, is that something that you would like, or you are not used to that?

Claire: Oh no, I'm. I like to pray dear, especially with someone that I know has the same sort of feeling, you know, you can tell, can't you?

Facilitator: Thank you Claire, that's lovely. Hetty, did you want to say anything about the power of prayer before we finish?

Hetty: Yes. I think about the, and I like to, to pray, and I think it helps, helps me.

(MacKinlay and Trevitt, 2012, p.251)

Actually getting to a church service was becoming more difficult for some of these people, as physical and mental issues complicated their ability to get to the services. Some had continued their connections with their last congregation, but it was becoming more difficult:

Facilitator: Hetty, did you want to say anything about the church services, anything, that's important to you at the moment?

Hetty: Well, more seem to be coming, don't they?

Daphne: Are you able to get anywhere these days, or can't you possible get anyway?

Hetty: Oh well.

Don: If someone takes you.

Hetty: Yes.

Daphne: Oh, sorry.

Hetty: Well I, I can't get anywhere.

Daphne: No you can't do it on your own, no.

Hetty: No.

Don: Neither can I, as a matter of fact, unless someone helps me, because I can't see very good.

Daphne: That's why I am very pleased that I can just take my walker thing and go in the lift and I am there. I can manage. I would not be able to go out on the street, and go to a different church, but I am very happy with this. Um, did you want to say something about the spiritual activities that you do, go to church, and things, and things that you do now, Hetty?

Hetty: No I, I didn't hear what you said love.

Facilitator: Would you like to say something about, um, how important going to church is for you?

Hetty: Yes. I enjoy it. And there seems to be a lot more going to, to the church, that's not much, is it?

Facilitator: Is there one part that you like particularly?

Hetty: Yeah, yes I like the, the…in the voice, I like the singing. I like the community singing too.

Facilitator: You do. You know a lot of songs, don't you?

(MacKinlay and Trevitt, 2012, pp.256–7)

Taking Communion or the Lord's Supper remained important for some:

Facilitator:	Communion, when you take Communion. What that means to you? How important it is?
Daphne:	Holy Communion, the bread and the wine, yes.
Hetty:	Well I, I feel different, having Communion.
Daphne:	Mmm.
Hetty:	I like it, I enjoy it.
Facilitator:	And, Claire, can you, do you want to say anything about taking Communion?
Claire:	No dear.
Facilitator:	That's okay.
Claire:	Except that it has always meant something to me, deep down inside, it is a feeling you can't explain.

(MacKinlay and Trevitt, 2012, pp.257–8)

Closure of session

This sixth session is the final of the six main weekly themes for spiritual reminiscence. If the weekly sessions are to continue, the same six themes are repeated. We have found that with people who have dementia, repeating these six themes benefits the participants over 24 weeks (or six months). Each round of sessions will elicit slightly different responses as the group members get to know each other better, and as they develop friendships with others in the group.

The long-term benefits of this spiritual reminiscence work include making new friends, more readily making connections in the small group settings and coming to a greater sense of meaning in their lives.

We stress that the communication in these group sessions is on emotions and spirituality, and importantly, not on cognition.

We have found consistently, throughout our work of more than a decade that people with dementia respond to meaningful conversation, even while they may be losing cognitive ability.

Bring the session to closure, re-emphasizing the positive aspects of the life journey. Thank the group members for sharing and encourage them to return for the next series of sessions, or if the whole 24 weeks have ended, then a similar small support group, perhaps focusing on other creative and pastoral activities may further assist in bonding connections between these people.

Reflection on the spiritual reminiscence process

The completion of the spiritual reminiscence groups, whether they were six or 24 weeks in length, provided a good opportunity to ask participants whether these were of benefit. In two of the 24 week research groups one of the participants died. In each group, there was the opportunity to remember the participant who had died and acknowledge their contribution to the group. In one instance, the wife of the deceased group member remained part of the same group. There she was able to gain comfort and support from the group as they remembered and talked about her husband.

Sometimes in residential facilities it is difficult for people to find opportunities to remember and talk about those who have died. At times staff will feel overburdened by a number of deaths occurring within their facility in a short period of time and find it hard to manage their own grief, let alone that of the residents. These groups gave an excellent opportunity for the participants to do grief work. The findings from the study also illustrated how both these group members were able to participate until within (in both cases) two weeks of their death.

You have now completed the spiritual reminiscence learning guide.

How would you go about planning your own program?

For additional information about reminiscence and spiritual reminiscence you may like to read MacKinlay and Trevitt (2012) *Finding Meaning in the Experience of Dementia: The Place of Spiritual Reminiscence Work,* London: Jessica Kingsley Publishers, or some of the other books included in the references list.

Appendix 1

Group topics for spiritual reminiscence

These are the weekly session topics, based on the MacKinlay Spiritual Tasks and Process of Ageing Model (2001) and used in a Linkage Grant 2002–2005. All pages in this appendix and Appendix 2 can be photocopied for your own use.

Topics for participants to explore their life journey

A series of six themes of broad questions can be used to facilitate the process of spiritual reminiscence over six weekly group sessions. The topics below are suggested outlines for guiding the themes for each weekly session.

Week 1: Life-meaning

- What gives greatest meaning to your life now? Follow up with questions like:
    - What is most important in your life?
    - What keeps you going?
    - Is life worth living?
    - If life is worth living – why is it worth living? If not, then you might like to ask – why do you feel like life is not worth living?
- Looking back over your life:
    - What do you remember with joy?
    - What do you remember with sadness?
    - What gives you greatest meaning to your life now?

Week 2: Relationships, isolation, connecting

- What are/have been the best things about relationships in your life?

Use this as a starting point for exploring relationships with the group.

Think of a number of questions, such as who visits you, who do you miss? Who have you been especially close to?

- Who visits you?

- Who do you miss?

- Who have you been especially close to?

- Do you have many friends here?

- Who are your friends?

- Do you ever feel lonely? When might you feel lonely? Follow up on things that might be associated with time of day, place etc.

- Do you like to be alone?

Week 3: Hopes, fears and worries

- What things do you worry about?

- Do you have any fears? What about?

- Do you feel you can talk to anyone about things that trouble you?

- What gives you hope now?

Week 4: Growing older and transcendence

- What's it like growing older?

- Do you have any health problems?

- Do you have memory problems? If so how does that affect what you want to do?

- What are the hardest things in your life now?

- Do you like living here? What's it like living here? Was it hard to settle in? (You can add other questions of a similar kind as appropriate.)

- As you reach the end of your life what do you hope for now?

- What do you look forward to?

Week 5: Spiritual and religious beliefs

- What do you think God is like?

- Do you have an image of God or some sense of a deity or otherness?

- If you hold an image of God, can you tell me about this image?

- Do you feel near to God?

- What are your earliest memories of church, mosque, temple or other worship?

- As a child, did you go to Sunday school, church or take part in any other religious or spiritual activities?

- Where do you go to get spiritual support?

- Who is the most important person to give you spiritual support?

- Do you find art or music expresses spirituality for you?

- Are plants and animals a way of expressing spirituality for you?

Week 6: Spiritual and religious practices

- Do you take part in any religious/spiritual activities now? For example, do you:

  - attend church services

  - take part in Bible studies

  - take part in other religious readings

  - pray

  - meditate or

  - attend study groups?

- Are there particular cultural and/or religious beliefs that should be considered in your care?

- How important are these to you?

- How can we help you to find meaning now?

Spiritual reminiscence and older people, a small group process

Information for intending participants, staff and families

Finding meaning in later life

A crucial task closely associated with hope, important for all people, and especially for older people, including those who have dementia.

Reminiscence

Reminiscence is essentially the process of remembering the past. Now widely used in aged care. Often it focuses on specific memory of event and enjoyment of these.

Spiritual reminiscence

This is a naturally occurring process for some older people that involves making sense and finding meaning of their lives. To be effective, it will go to the core of deepest meaning in the person's life. In the twentieth century, we had largely lost the skills of spiritual reminiscence. Now we are realizing just how important our individual stories are; for the person whose story it is, for their families, and when in residential care, for the staff to be able to give best care.

The use of small group reminiscence for people who have dementia

Spiritual reminiscence is a way of telling a life story with an emphasis on what gives meaning to life, what has given joy or brought sadness. This process can be simply a natural process of ageing; it may be done on a one-on-one basis of pastoral care, or it may be done as a small group process. There is the added value with small group work of facilitating the formation of new friendships. When small group work is done it makes better use of time, more people can take part and fewer facilitators are needed. It also encourages unique interactions between participants. They enjoy each other's stories and experiences. Listening to others triggers their own memories and enhances participation in the discussion. Participants lend each other support and comfort. In some cases this process may encourage 'rementia' (Sixsmith, Stilwell and Copeland, 1993) when communication may seem to increase, in a supported environment.

This group will be run each week, for a maximum of about an hour. We have found with our work that once the participants get to know each other they make new friends and this takes longer for those with dementia due to their communication challenges.

Aim of the small groups at (name of organization or facility)

This small group will be facilitated by (insert name of facilitator). It will introduce the process to (insert name of place), and also be an opportunity of training for (insert name of facility) staff to equip them to conduct further groups into the future that may become part of the offerings provided by the facility.

References

Abdalla, M. and Patel, I. (2010) An Islamic Perspective on Ageing and Spirituality. In E. MacKinlay (ed.) *Ageing and Spirituality Across Faith and Cultures*. London: Jessica Kingsley Publishers.

Access Economics (2006) *Listen Hear! The Economic Impact and Cost of Hearing Loss in Australia*. Canberra: Access Economics.

Access Economics (2009) *Keeping Dementia Front of Mind: Incidence and Prevalence 2009–2050*. Executive Summary. Canberra: Access Economics.

Allen, N. H., Burns, A., Newton, V., Hickson, F. *et al.* (2003) 'The effects of improving hearing in dementia.' *Age and Ageing, 32*, 2, 189–93.

Alzheimer's Disease Research (2011) Available at www.ahaf.org/alzheimers/about/understanding/facts.html, accessed on 10 May 2013.

Alzeihmer's Society (2011) Statistics. Available at www.alzehimers.org.uk, accessed on 10 May 2013.

Australian Institute of Health and Welfare (2012) *Dementia in Australia*. Cat. No. AGE 70. Canberra: AIHW.

Barzaghi, S. (2010) The Spiritual Needs of the Aged and Dying: A Buddhist Perspective. In E. MacKinlay (ed.) *Ageing and Spirituality Across Faith and Cultures*. London: Jessica Kingsley Publishers.

Behuniak, S. (2011) 'The living dead? The construction of those living with Alzheimer's as zombies.' *Ageing and Society, 31*, 70–92.

Berk, R. (2010) 'The active ingredients in humor: Psychological benefits and risks for older adults.' *Educational Gerontology, 27*, 3, 323–39.

Bird, M. (2002) Dementia and Suffering in Nursing Homes. In E. MacKinlay (ed.) *Mental Health and Spirituality in Later Life*. New York: Haworth Press.

Bryden, C. (2005) *Dancing with Dementia: My Story of Living Positively with Dementia*. London: Jessica Kingsley Publishers.

Bryden, C. (2012) *Who will I Be when I Die?* London: Jessica Kingsley Publishers.

Bryden, C. and MacKinlay, E. B. (2002) 'Dementia – A Spiritual journey towards the divine: A personal view of dementia.' *Journal of Religious Gerontology, 13*, 3/4, 69–75.

Burgoon, J. K. and Bacue, A. (2003) Nonverbal Communication Skills. In B. R. Burleson and J. O. Greene (eds) *Handbook of Communication and Social Interaction Skills*. Mahwah, NJ: Erlbaum.

Butler, R. (1995) Foreword. In B. Haight and J. Webster. (eds) *The Art and Science of Reminiscing*. Washington: Taylor and Francis.

Butler, R. N. (1963) The life review: An interpretation of Reminiscence in the Aged. In B. L. Neugarten (ed.) (1968) *Middle Age and Aging: A reader in social psychology*. Chicago, IL: The University of Chicago Press.

Byrne, L. and MacKinlay, E. (2012) 'Seeking meaning: Making art and the experience of spirituality in dementia care.' *Journal of Religion, Spirituality and Aging, 25*, 1–2, 105–19.

Chiu, M. J., Chen, T., Yip, P., Hua, M. and Tang, L. (2006) 'Behavioural and psychotic symptoms on different types of dementia.' *Journal Formosa Medical Association, 105*, 7, 556–62.

Cohen, J. (2010) From Ageing to Sage-ing: Judiasm and Ageing. In E. MacKinlay (ed.) *Ageing and Spirituality Across Faiths and Cultures*. London: Jessica Kingsley Publishers.

Coleman, P. G. (1999) 'Creating a life story: The task of reconciliation.' *The Gerontologist, 39*, 2, 133–39.

de Medeiros, K. (2014) *Narrative Gerontology in Research and Practice*. New York, NY: Springer Publishing Company.

De Baggio, T. (2003) *Losing my mind: An intimate look at life with Alzheimers*. New York, NY: The Free Press.

Ekman, S., Norberg, A., Viitanen, M. and Winbald, B. (1991) 'Care of demented patients with severe communication problems.' *Scandinavian Journal of Caring Science, 5*, 3, 163–70.

Emre, M., Aarsland, D., Brown, R., Burn, D., *et al.* (2007) 'Clinical diagnostic criteria for dementia associated with Parkinson's disease.' *Movement Disorders, 22*, 12, 1689–707.

Erikson, E. H., Erikson, J. M. and Kivnick, H. Q. (1986) *Vital Involvement in Old Age.* New York, NY: W. W. Norton and Co.

Ferri, C., Prince, M., Brayne, C., Brodaty, H. *et al.* (2005) 'Global prevalence of dementia: A Delphi consensus study.' *The Lancet, 366*, 9503, 2112–17.

George, D. (2010) 'Overcoming the social death of dementia through language.' *The Lancet, 376*, 9741, 586–7.

Gibson, F. (1998) *Reminiscence and Recall: A Guide to Good Practice.* London: Age Concern.

Gibson, F. (2004) *The Past in the Present: Using Reminiscence in Health and Social Care.* Baltimore, MD: Health Professions Press Ltd.

Goldsmith, M. (1996) *Hearing the Voice of People with Dementia: Opportunities and Obstacles.* London: Jessica Kingsley Publishers.

Goldsmith, M. (2004) *In a Strange Land: People with Dementia and the Local Church.* Nottingham: 4M Publications.

Herman, R. and Williams, K. (2009) 'Elderspeak's influence on resistiveness to care: Focus on behavioral events.' *America Journal of Alzheimer's Disease and Other Dementias, 24*, 417–22.

Hubbard, G., Cook, A., Tester, S. and Downs, M. (2002) 'Beyond words: Older people with dementia using and interpreting non-verbal behaviour.' *Journal of Ageing Studies, 16*, 115–167.

Hughes, J. C., Louw, S. J. and Sabat, S. R. (eds) (2006) *Dementia, Mind, Meaning, and the Person.* Oxford: Oxford University Press.

Kenyon, G. M. 'Telling and listening to stories: Creating a wisdom environment for older people'. *Generations, 27*, 3, 30–33.

Kenyon, G. M., Clark, P. and de Vries, B. (eds) (2001) *Narrative Gerontology: Theory, Research, and Practice.* New York, NY: Springer.

Killick, J. (1997) *You are Words: Dementia Poems.* London: Journal of Dementia Care.

Killick, J. (2004) Dementia, Identity and Spirituality. In E. MacKinlay (ed.) *Spirituality of Later Life: On Humor and Despair.* New York, NY: Haworth Press.

Killick, J. (2006) Helping the Flame to Stay Bright: Celebrating the Spiritual in Dementia. In E. MacKinlay (ed.) *Aging, Spirituality and Palliative Care.* New York, NY: Haworth Press.

Killick, J. and Allan, K. (2001) *Communication and the Care of Older People with Dementia.* Buckinghamshire: Open University Press.

Kimble, M. (2004) 'Human despair and comic transcendence.' *Journal of Religious Gerontology, 16*, 3, 1–11.

Kitwood, T. (1993) 'Person and process in dementia.' Editorial. *International Journal of Geriatric Psychiatry, 8*, 541–5.

Kitwood, T. (1997) *Dementia Reconsidered.* Buckinghamshire: Open University Press.

Kovach, S. and Robinson, J. (1996) 'The room-mate relationship for the elderly nursing home resident.' *Journal of Social and Personal Relationships, 13*, 4, 627–34.

MacEvoy, P., Eden, J. and Plant, R. (2014) 'Dementia communication using empathetic curiosity.' *The Nursing Times, 110*, 24, 12–15.

MacKinlay, E. (2001) *The Spiritual Dimension of Ageing.* London: Jessica Kingsley Publishers.

MacKinlay, E. (2006) *Spiritual Growth and Care in the Fourth Age of Life.* London: Jessica Kingsley Publishers.

MacKinlay, E. (2012) *Palliative Care, Ageing and Spirituality.* London: Jessica Kingsley Publishers.

MacKinlay, E. and Burns, R. (2013) Age-related life-changing events and baby boomer spirituality. An unpublished research project for UnitingCare Ageing. NSW: ACT.

MacKinlay, E. and Trevitt, C. (2005) Finding meaning in the experience of dementia: The place of spiritual reminiscence work. Unpublished report to ARC – Linkage Grant.

MacKinlay, E. and Trevitt, C. (2006) *Spiritual Reminiscence for Older People with Dementia: A Learning Package.* Canberra: CAPS.

MacKinlay, E. and Trevitt, C. (2012) *Finding Meaning in the Experience of Dementia: The Place of Spiritual Reminiscence Work.* London: Jessica Kingsley Publishers.

MacKinlay, E., McDonald, T. and Niven, A. (2011) Minimising the impact of depression and dementia for elders in residential care. Unpublished Research report. Canberra: CAPS. (Funded by J.O. and J.R. Wicking Trust.)

MacKinlay, K. (2001) Listening to people with dementia: A pastoral care perspective. Conference presentation: Mental Health and Spirituality. National Conference, Centre for Ageing and Pastoral Studies, Canberra, 21–24 September 2001. Unpublished report.

Martin, R. (2009) Humour. In S. Lopez (ed.) *The Encyclopedia of Positive Psychology.* Oxford: Wiley-Blackwell.

Matsumoto, Y. (2009) 'Dealing with life changes: Humour in painful self-disclosures by elderly Japanese women.' *Ageing and Society, 29,* 929–52.

Moody, H. R. (1995) Mysticism. In M. A. Kimble, S. H. McFadden, J. W. Ellor and J. J. Seeber (eds) *Aging, Spirituality, and Religion: A Handbook.* Minneapolis, MN: Augsburg Fortress Press.

Mukerdam, N. and Livingstone, G. (2012) 'Reducing the stigma associated with dementia: Approaches and goals.' *Aging Health, 8,* 4, 377–86.

Naue, U. and Kroll, T. (2008) '*The demented other: Identity and difference in dementia.*' *Nursing Philosophy, 10,* 1, 26–33.

Porter, H. (2002) The long goodbyew. *Dementia in Scotland newsletter.* Issue 38, 7.

Post, G. (2006) 'Respectare': Moral Respect for the Lives of the Deeply Forgetful. In J. C. Hughes, S. J. Louw, and S. R. Sabat (eds) *Dementia Mind, Meaning, and the Person.* Oxford: Oxford University Press.

Randall, W. L. and Kenyon, G. M. (2004) 'Time, story, and wisdom: Emerging themes in narrative gerontology.' *Canadian Journal on Aging, 23,* 4, 333–46.

Rayner, A. and Bilimoria, P. (2010) Dying: An Approach to Care from Hindu and Buddhist Perspectives. In E. MacKinlay (ed.) *Ageing and Spirituality Across Faiths and Cultures.* London: Jessica Kingsley Publishers.

Sixsmith, A., Stilwell, J. and Copeland, J. (1993) 'Rementia': Challenging the Limits of Dementia Care. *International Journal of Geriatric Psychiatry, 8,* 12, 993–1000.

Smith, M. and Buckwalter, K. (2005) 'Behaviours associated with dementia.' *American Journal of Nursing, 105,* 7, 40–52.

Snowden, D. (2001) *Ageing with Grace.* London: Harper Collins.

Stokes, G. (2010) *And Still the Music Plays.* London: Hawker Publications.

Trevitt, C. and MacKinlay, E. (2006) '"I am just an ordinary person…" Spiritual reminiscence in older people with memory loss.' *Journal of Religion, Spirituality and Aging, 19,* 2/3, 77–89.

Webster, J. and Haight, B. (2002) *Critical Advances in Reminiscence Work.* New York, NY: Springer Publishing Company.

Williams, K., Herman, R., Gajewski, B. and Wilson, K. (2009) 'Elderspeak communication: Impact on dementia care.' *American Journal of Alzheimer's Disease and other Dementias, 24,* 11, 11–20.

Woods, R. (1989) *Alheimer's Disease: Coping with a living death.* London: Souvenir.

Index

Sub-headings in *italics* indicate figures.